Sourcebook for Receptive and Expressive Language Functioning

Beaumont®
William Beaumont Hospital

William Beaumont Hospital
Speech and Language Pathology Series

Series Editors
Michael I. Rolnick, Ph.D.
William Beaumont Hospital

Alex Johnson, Ph.D.
Wayne State University

A complete listing of the books in this series can be found online at wsupress.wayne.edu

Sourcebook for Receptive and Expressive Language Functioning

Susan Howell Brubaker, M.S., CCC-SLP

Wayne State University Press
Detroit, Michigan

Manufactured in the United States of America.
10 09 08 07 06 5 4 3 2 1

ISBN: 0-8143-3314-1

∞ The paper used in this publication meets the minimum requirements of the American National Standard for Information Sciences—Permanence of Paper for Printed Library Materials, ANSI Z39.48-1984.

CONTENTS

ABOUT THE AUTHOR

Susan Howell Brubaker is Assistant Director of the Speech and Language Pathology Department at William Beaumont Hospital, Royal Oak, Michigan. For more than thirty years, she has specialized in working with adults who have suffered communicative loss as a result of neurological dysfunction or brain injury. She holds the B.S. from St. Lawrence University, Canton, New York, the M.S. from Ithaca College, Ithaca, New York, and the Certificate of Clinical Competence from the American Speech-Language-Hearing Association. She is the recipient of the Distinguished Service Award from the Michigan Speech-Language-Hearing Association (MSHA).

My colleagues Carolyn A. Doty, M.A., CCC-SLP, Supervisor of Outpatient Adult Services, and Lisa M. Mammoser, M.A., CCC-SLP, Coordinator of the Outpatient Diagnostic Program, worked many hours on the plan and composition of this book. Their excellent clinical sensibilities ensured the content was functional and the organization was both clinician- and patient-friendly. As always, their perceptive input, advice, humor, and ideas throughout any project are most valued.

I want to acknowledge Kristin Harpster Lawrence, Managing Editor of Wayne State University Press, for her thoughtful guidance and concern with the integrity of this project. I am grateful to Kristin for her calm and straightforward approach on this sourcebook and the other revised workbooks as well as all of the other detail work she performed to ensure the professional look and functionality of the books.

OTHER BOOKS BY SUSAN HOWELL BRUBAKER

Other Susan Howell Brubaker books published by Wayne State University Press:

Sourcebook for Speech, Language, and Cognition: Stimulus Materials for Rehabilitation, Books 1, 2, and 3

Workbook for Cognitive Skills: Exercises for Thought Processing and Word Retrieval

Workbook for Language Skills: Exercises for Written and Verbal Expression

Workbook for Aphasia: Exercises for Expressive and Receptive Language Functioning

Basic Level Workbook for Aphasia

Workbook for Reasoning Skills: Exercises for Functional Reasoning and Reading Comprehension

INTRODUCTION

The *Sourcebook for Receptive and Expressive Language Functioning* is a comprehensive resource of stimulus questions for you to draw upon for clients or patients from upper elementary to geriatric age. If you have used my *Sourcebooks for Speech, Language, and Cognition,* the format and diagnostic divider pages of this book will be familiar to you.

The *Sourcebook for Receptive and Expressive Language Functioning* was written for adults and adolescents with acquired impairments resulting from neurological dysfunction, disease, and injury. Speech pathologists report the *Sourcebooks'* versatility and also use them with a much younger and diverse population, including those with stuttering, autism spectrum disorders, ESL, and central auditory processing and other disorders. As a creative clinician, you will find great flexibility and many uses for this volume. The goal is to provide busy clinicians with a huge collection of questions that are current, real-life, and humorous; vocabulary that is relevant, functional, and interesting; and topics that are thought-provoking, diverse, and personal. Additional care was taken to ensure that questions have great variety in vocabulary, concepts, terms, and ideas. It is this clinician's experience that it is easier to take more difficult material and scale it down than it is to make easier material more difficult.

There are a number of features that make this *Sourcebook* unique and user-friendly.

- The book is divided into two sections clearly defined by colored tabs. The six purple tabs represent receptive comprehension skills and the six gray tabs represent verbal / nonverbal expressive skills.
- The unique tabbed pages function as more than divider pages. When you open to a divider page, you will see listed the names of all exercises in that target area along with the first question from each one. This page serves as a diagnostic screening tool and hierarchy of tasks to help you determine a patient's level of ability. For each of the screening questions, the numbered page has 20 follow-up practice questions of that same type. This diagnostic process can be used within one target area or across all receptive and expressive divider areas.
- The hard cover, heavier divider pages, and lay-flat spiral binding make the *Sourcebook* sturdy, durable, and long-lasting.
- Since this is not a patient workbook, the print is smaller so most exercises fit on one page. This allows you to scan the questions more easily. The added white space gives you room to personalize the book by adding your own notes, answers, or additional questions.
- All of the 296 exercises have 20 items so that percentages and outcomes can be easily determined. The receptive (purple) and expressive (gray) divisions and all target areas start with easier activities and progress to more complex materials. Within each target area, exercises are in a general order by type and by difficulty.
- The *Sourcebook* is a resource and not a step-by-step program. It offers flexibility for you to modify the type and difficulty level of stimulus and response items. You can be creative in what you present, how you present it, and how you build on the response.
- An answer key is not included for two reasons. First, only the Functional Math section has right/wrong answers and only a few exercises in the Naming target area are tricky. If you wish to have those answers available, there is room to write them on the page. The second reason is that each answer should be assessed on its own merits. If an answer is not conventional, let the patient explain or defend it. Individuals can give you important data by their answer, inter-

pretation, or even non-answer (as in the one we all hear: *I never did/knew/had to deal with that*). You might accept answers early in treatment that you would not accept with the same exercise at a later date. Assessing answers can help you plan treatment, develop strategies, goals, and self-monitoring. Preconceived answers may stifle creativity and cognitive flexibility on the part of both the patient and the clinician.

- The introduction to the target areas below suggests some ways that the exercises can be modified to become easier or more difficult depending on what is needed. The creative clinician will, no doubt, find even more ways to use them.

Receptive Language Functioning (purple tabs)

Yes / No questions—35 exercises. This target area starts with simple orientation and proceeds to longer and more complex exercises. Yes / no questions are easy to modify into true / false, multiple-choice, or open-ended (naming) questions thus providing the means to expand the use of the exercises. To add more complexity, add another element to the question or ask "Was the last question about . . ." adding an element of recall.

Multiple Choice questions—27 exercises. Most of the multiple choice exercises have two answer choices within the question. Questions can be made easier by changing them to true / false or yes / no. Questions can be made more difficult by adding another choice, or by rewording the question so it becomes open-ended (naming) or requiring a sentence answer.

Sentence Comprehension questions—26 exercises. These exercises range from simple one-step directions to exercises with up to 10 elements. Omitting or adding information to the question can manipulate the difficulty level. Exercises in which there are statements followed by comprehension questions can be modified by how general or specific the question is, and whether it is yes / no, open-ended, or requires repetition of some part of the original statement.

Basic Math problems—16 exercises. These exercises are mainly computation or "mental math." A few exercises were included to cover cost awareness, common number facts, and conversions. The questions can be made easier or harder as needed.

Functional Material—20 exercises. The exercises in this target area are arranged by type of material, not by difficulty level. You need to have everyday items such as a newspaper or pill bottle available. The patient answers questions about the item. You can add or change questions by type and difficulty depending on your needs and the materials used.

Paragraphs with comprehension questions—17 exercises. This target area contains paragraphs of varying length and complexity with one or more comprehension questions. The questions are a combination of yes / no, multiple choice, or short answer and can be modified according to your needs. Some elements of the sentence can be omitted or other points can be included. Additional comprehension questions can be easily added.

Expressive Language Functioning (gray tabs)

Nonverbal Communication—15 exercises. These exercises aim to build communication through drawing, gestures, and pantomime as well as to develop a means of functional communication. The exercises also are practice in using these methods to express wants and needs. Other nonverbal responses such as writing or use of electronic devices can be used not only with this target area but with questions throughout the book. These exercises can also be used by those with emerging speech.

Completions—24 exercises. Completions are a familiar technique to cue words and automatic speech, and as a means of eliciting speech at a word and phrase level. While most of the questions can be completed with a single word, they can be modified so the individual must generate a phrase. Modifications to increase difficulty include requiring more than one answer or having the patient repeat the whole question.

Naming—32 exercises. Naming tasks especially with picture cards are common. These exercises range in type and difficulty to challenge from emerging to high-level naming. The exercises can be made easier by making the category easier or by giving hints for a specific answer. The difficulty level can be increased by requiring multiple answers—making them Word Fluency tasks or by adding parameters to the question.

Word Fluency—28 exercises. Word Fluency exercises are naming tasks that require more than one answer. With multiple answers, there is more room for interpretation, creativity, and flexibility in a response. But for some this makes the task more difficult. The exercises can be made easier by omitting some parameters or making it a naming task (previous target area) by requiring only one answer. Additional challenges could be to require a higher number of answers or answers that begin with a certain letter.

Sentence Formulation—29 exercises. The directions for these exercises require creating a simple or complex sentence as a response. The first ten exercises provide words or phrases to incorporate into a sentence. The remaining exercises require not only the construction of a sentence but carefully considered content. The exercises can be made easier by accepting a nonverbal response, or a word or phrase rather than sentence. They can be made more difficult by having the patient include other points, expand a response, or by you asking follow-up questions. Most exercises in this target area can be interchanged with that of Longer Answers.

Longer Answers—27 exercises. In this target area, the patient is asked to construct either a complex sentence and/or multiple sentences with multiple bits of information. Each exercise presents questions that may trigger follow-up questions or discussion. Many of the responses can be insightful, personal, and intriguing. The difficulty level can be modified by requiring more or less information, or shorter answers that do not need to be in a sentence.

YES / NO

17 Personal Orientation ....*Is your first name ___________ ?*

18 Time Orientation........................*Is it daytime / night?*

19 Personal Questions ....*Are you left-handed?*

20 Basic Feasibility ....*Can you grow wings?*

21 Basic Categories ....*Is a Cadillac a car?*

22 Basic Single Elements ....*Can bones break?*

23 Single Elements ....*Are thermometers flexible?*

24 Basic Meanings..........................*Is a bedpan a cooking utensil?*

25 Parts ....*Is flannel used in shirts?*

26 Brand Names ....*Does Vlasic make pickles?*

27 Visuals.......................................*Does a skunk have a long tail?*

28 Safety Factors ....*Should you step quickly into a hot shower?*

29 Function ....*Is a blowtorch used to dry hair?*

30 Meanings...................................*Does a barricade keep you away from something?*

31 Usage ....*Could you use a calculator to figure a tip?*

32 Terms ....*Is a litterbug an insect?*

33 Famous People...........................*Is Vincent Van Gogh known for being an artist?*

34 Human Qualities ....*Is an organized person usually neat?*

35 Decisions...................................*If it is Sunday, is it a weekend?*

36 All or Some................................*Do all plants need sunlight to grow?*

37 Feasibility ....*Can a fire alarm go off when there isn't a fire?*

38 Necessity...................................*Do you need a zip code to call long distance?*

39 Mixed Questions........................*Could you daydream at night?*

40 Judgment Calls ....*Would you spend time in a barn if you were allergic to hay?*

41 Comparisons ....*Is chicken broth thinner than beef stew?*

42 Dimensions ....*Are your toes longer than your fingers?*

43 Figures of Speech ....*Do you need a pencil to draw a blank?*

44 Emotions ....*Are you bored if a lecture is motivating?*

45 Estimates...................................*Does an elevator hold more people than a bus?*

46 Two Variables ....*Can a food be both cold and spicy?*

47 Three Variables ....*Are cardinals and hawks both birds?*

48 Complex Vocabulary ....*If a warranty expired, would it be valid?*

49 Linked Questions........................*Can you wear a sock on either foot? Can you wear a shoe on either foot?*

50 Multiple Variables......................*Are oysters and octopuses both saltwater shellfish?*

51 Subject Questions ....*Think about an oil painting. Could it increase in value? Could it burn? Could it be framed?*

Directions: Insert or choose a word based on your information. Answer the questions with yes or no.

1. Is your first name _________ ?
2. Is your last name _________ ?
3. (city) Do you live in _________ ?
4. (state) Do you live in _________ ?
5. (street) Do you live on _________ ?
6. Do you live alone?
7. (marital status) Are you _________ ?
8. (living situation) Do you live in a(n) _________ ?
9. (family) Do you have brothers or sisters?
10. (spouse name) Is your wife/husband's name _________ ?
11. (age) Are you _________ years old?
12. (birthday month) Is your birthday in _________ ?
13. Do you have children?
14. (number) Do you have _________ children / grandchildren?
15. Do you have a pet?
16. (accompanying person name) Is this _________ ?
17. (accompanying person) Did _________ bring you today?
18. (name of location) Right now are you in _________ ?
19. (glasses, hearing aid) Are you wearing _________ ?
20. (medical condition) Did you have a _________ ?

Time Orientation

Receptive: Yes / No

Directions: Insert or choose a word based on your information. Answer the question with yes or no.

1. Is it daytime / night?
2. Is it morning / afternoon / evening?
3. Is it Monday / Tuesday / Wednesday / Thursday / Friday?
4. Is it the weekend?
5. (any holiday) Is it _________ today?
6. Is it around (breakfast / lunch / dinner) time?
7. Have you eaten (breakfast / lunch / dinner) today?
8. (season) Is it _________ ?
9. (weather) Is it _________ outside?
10. (year of birth) Were you born in the year _________ ?
11. (current month) Are we in the month of _________ ?
12. Is it near the end of the month?
13. Is it almost time for you to go to bed?
14. Do you usually go to bed around 11:00?
15. Have we been talking for about an hour?
16. (year) Is it the year _________ ?
17. (medical condition) Has it been more than a year since you had _________ ?
18. (appointment time) Was your appointment at _________ ?
19. Is today your birthday?
20. Are you alone right now?

Directions: When indicated, insert or choose a word based on your information. Answer the questions with yes or no.

1. Are you left-handed?
2. Are you standing up?
3. Are you taller than your father?
4. Do you have any cavities in your teeth?
5. Are you wearing a watch?
6. Do you have brown hair?
7. Is your hair longer than you usually wear it?
8. Are you an only child?
9. Do you use a wheelchair / cane?
10. Do you have pierced ears / tattoos?
11. Do you like to drink tea?
12. Were you the oldest child in your family?
13. Are you taller than five feet?
14. Have you been married more than _________ years?
15. Do you have blue eyes?
16. Have you been in your current home longer than _________ years?
17. Were you born in this state?
18. Do you speak another language besides English?
19. Do you watch a lot of television?
20. Is there a window in this room?

Basic Feasibility

Receptive: Yes / No

Directions: Answer the questions with yes or no.

1. Can you grow wings?
2. Can you run in an orchard?
3. Can you sing a melody?
4. Can you peel a strawberry?
5. Can you memorize a joke?
6. Can you lose a passport?
7. Can you throw a closet?
8. Can you refill a glass?
9. Can you slip on fog?
10. Can you take a nap?
11. Can you hear a rumor?
12. Can you dig with a needle?
13. Can you make a bed?
14. Can you break a record?
15. Can you lay an egg?
16. Can you kick a stone?
17. Can you wear a slipcover?
18. Can you carry a dream?
19. Can you climb a ladder?
20. Can you drive through a tunnel?

Directions: Answer the questions with yes or no.

1. Is a Cadillac a car?
2. Is brass a color?
3. Are marigolds a flower?
4. Is a night crawler a piece of furniture?
5. Is a six-pack a weapon?
6. Is basketball a sport?
7. Is a cocker spaniel a bird?
8. Is a pork chop a type of meat?
9. Is poker a card game?
10. Is yogurt a beverage?
11. Is July a day of the week?
12. Is a maple a type of tree?
13. Is Berlin a country?
14. Is a gorilla an animal?
15. Is a turtle an insect?
16. Is a shoulder a part of your body?
17. Is Scorpio a planet?
18. Is Wyoming a state?
19. Is Cornell a university?
20. Is a chicken potpie a dessert?

Directions: Answer the questions with yes or no.

1. Can bones break?
2. Do dishes melt?
3. Can squirrels swim?
4. Do doors open?
5. Can juice freeze?
6. Can shadows sing?
7. Do planes fly?
8. Does chalk grow?
9. Do almonds have shells?
10. Do mugs have wings?
11. Are diamonds expensive?
12. Can opinions change?
13. Do rubber bands stretch?
14. Does soup melt?
15. Are yield signs red?
16. Do candles burn?
17. Do fish have fur?
18. Can pipes crack?
19. Does moss grow?
20. Is caramel sour?

Directions: Answer the questions with yes or no.

1. Are thermometers flexible?
2. Is foil transparent?
3. Do inner tubes float?
4. Does mahogany sting?
5. Is chalk edible?
6. Can wallpaper peel?
7. Do bears hibernate?
8. Is sandpaper slippery?
9. Can a boat capsize?
10. Are fences fragile?
11. Does mold grow?
12. Is digestion automatic?
13. Are allergies greasy?
14. Do sequins sparkle?
15. Can warranties expire?
16. Does concrete evaporate?
17. Do billboards advertise?
18. Are magnets sticky?
19. Are belts adjustable?
20. Is glue nutritious?

Basic Meanings

Receptive: Yes / No

Directions: Answer the questions with yes or no.

1. Is a bedpan a cooking utensil?
2. Is a maze a type of puzzle?
3. Are shingles a covering for windows?
4. Is a trophy an award for doing something well?
5. Does an adoption happen when a marriage ends?
6. Is a raisin a dried grape?
7. Is a swamp a dry area of land?
8. Is a pier a place that lets you walk out over water?
9. Are earmuffs a type of hearing aid?
10. Is a pantry a place to keep food?
11. Do tonsils help you digest food?
12. Is a pension a writing utensil?
13. Is tapioca similar to pudding?
14. Is a glacier a mountain of ice?
15. Are Brussels sprouts small trees?
16. Is a razor used to carve meat?
17. Is jazz a type of music?
18. Are matzo balls used in sports?
19. Is a fairy tale a true story?
20. Do antlers grow on some animals?

Directions: Answer the questions with yes or no.

1. Is flannel used in shirts?
2. Are rafters used in houses?
3. Are paddles used on sleds?
4. Is yeast used in bread?
5. Are feathers used in omelets?
6. Are rules used in a contest?
7. Are hammocks used in bedrooms?
8. Are filters used in vacuums?
9. Are concession stands used in stadiums?
10. Are wood chips used in pillows?
11. Is spandex used in clothing?
12. Are quilts used on beds?
13. Are passports used in restaurants?
14. Is straw used in a barn?
15. Is garlic used in aspirin?
16. Is gas used in motorcycles?
17. Is leather used in ovens?
18. Is ink used in lamps?
19. Are strings used on guitars?
20. Are dice used in games?

Brand Names

Receptive Yes / No

Directions: Answer the questions with yes or no.

1. Does Vlasic make pickles?
2. Does Sunbeam make shampoo?
3. Does Hallmark make carpets?
4. Does Godiva make chocolate?
5. Does Arm & Hammer make tools?
6. Does Ever-Ready make batteries?
7. Does Fruit of the Loom make wine?
8. Does Pillsbury make pasta?
9. Does Quaker make oatmeal?
10. Does Reebok make HDTV's?
11. Does Kenmore make appliances?
12. Does Oreck make furniture?
13. Does Michelob make wine?
14. Does DiGiorno make pizza?
15. Does Velveeta make pudding?
16. Does Butterball produce turkeys?
17. Does Ragu make ketchup?
18. Does Snapple make canned fruit?
19. Does Grey Poupon make mustard?
20. Does Crisco make ice cream?

Directions: Answer the questions with yes or no.

1. Does a skunk have a long tail?
2. Does a nickel have an eagle on it?
3. Does a stove usually have four burners?
4. Is an exit sign usually green?
5. Does a touch-tone phone have 12 buttons?
6. Do you twist off the top of a soft drink can?
7. Is Neopolitan ice cream more than two colors?
8. Is eggplant green?
9. Is a knife sharp on two sides?
10. Is a blanket hemmed on all four sides?
11. On a keyboard, is the *Enter* key on the left?
12. On a light switch, is the switch down in the off position?
13. Do dice have six sides?
14. Do mice have long ears?
15. Is the skin on an onion wrinkled?
16. Is a book's binding on the left as you look at it?
17. Are there seven columns on a bingo card?
18. Is a paper clip pointed?
19. Do you put a key in a door on the right side?
20. Can you see through Saran Wrap?

Safety Factors

Receptive: Yes / No

Directions: Answer the questions with yes or no.

1. Should you step quickly into a hot shower?
2. Should you lean over a balcony to see below?
3. Should you have an extra supply of batteries on hand?
4. Should you move a power line that has fallen across your path?
5. Should you throw out a used tissue?
6. Should you drink water from a lake?
7. Should you get an X-ray for a cold sore / fever blister?
8. Should you keep your toenails trimmed?
9. Should you race a motorcycle over a dirt and gravel road?
10. Should you wear bright clothing when you go hunting?
11. Should you walk barefoot in the dark?
12. Should you write your social security number on a check?
13. Should you slice away from yourself with a knife?
14. Should you drive after dark if you have poor night vision?
15. Should you salt your food before you taste it?
16. Should you wear a seat belt if you are a passenger in a car?
17. Should you light a match if you smell gas?
18. Should you mow a lawn in sandals?
19. Should you take small bites of food and eat slowly?
20. Should you use hot plates to take a pan out of the oven?

Directions: Answer the questions with yes or no.

1. Is a blowtorch used to dry hair?
2. Is a paddle used to beat an egg?
3. Is construction paper used in building a house?
4. Are thumbtacks used to repair a hem?
5. Is a remote control used to operate something from a distance?
6. Is an emery board used to file nails?
7. Is a nutcracker used to shell a peanut?
8. Is a chairlift used to take people up a mountain?
9. Is a pacemaker used to measure distance?
10. Is a crane used in constructing high-rise buildings?
11. Is a chisel used to cut metal?
12. Is a CAT scan used by people?
13. Is a receipt used to get a refund?
14. Is a magnet used to stick things on metal?
15. Is a sledgehammer used to hang a large picture?
16. Is a cleaver used to cut meat?
17. Is a squash racket used to kill bugs?
18. Is a corkscrew used to open a bottle of champagne?
19. Is insulin used to regulate sugar levels in blood?
20. Is steel wool used in clothing designs?

Meanings

Receptive: Yes / No

Directions: Answer the questions with yes or no.

1. Does a barricade keep you away from something?
2. If something is laminated, is it covered in paint?
3. Is a limerick a type of poem?
4. Does tuition involve the exchange of money?
5. Could a man's voice be described as a baritone?
6. Is a layover something you get from sleeping too much?
7. Is confetti used at celebrations?
8. Is dermatology the study of plants?
9. Is a monogram formed from initials?
10. Is a siesta a type of Spanish home?
11. Is your signature your autograph?
12. Is a ransom a type of investment?
13. Are some truffles made from chocolate?
14. Is a slalom race done on snow?
15. Is plaque a protective coating on your teeth?
16. Is a scandal something to aspire to?
17. Is a banister a type of stair railing?
18. Is a whimper a quiet noise?
19. Does a viral infection cause allergies?
20. Is a dolly used to move boxes?

Directions: Answer the questions with yes or no.

1. Could you use a calculator to figure a tip?
2. Are close-captioned TV shows helpful to blind people?
3. Would you get a pedicure to cure acne?
4. Do arteries carry blood through the body?
5. Does dry ice keep things from being mildewed?
6. Would a man buy a condominium for birth control?
7. Would you check an emblem to get information about a product?
8. Would you put chlorine in a pool to kill bacteria?
9. Would a laxative help cure laryngitis?
10. Could you use a shower cap in the rain?
11. Would you go to a flea market to get a bargain?
12. Is a placebo a cure for an illness?
13. Would you use a snorkel to scuba dive?
14. Is Chapstick used to clean leather?
15. Would you get a DVD player to watch movies at home?
16. Are olives usually part of an antipasto?
17. Would you take an aphrodisiac for a headache?
18. Is acupuncture used to prevent meats from spoiling?
19. Is a septic tank a place to store waste material?
20. Is an antihistamine used to prevent diabetes?

Terms

Receptive: Yes / No

Directions: Answer the questions with yes or no.

1. Is a litterbug an insect?
2. Can people eat animal crackers?
3. Can you wear cotton candy?
4. Would you like a clean bill of health?
5. Would you bring food to a potluck supper?
6. Do you sit at a table of contents?
7. Can you use a lawn chair on a deck?
8. Would you take pills for growing pains?
9. Can you talk into an answering machine?
10. Do you study for a blood test?
11. Do you get wet at a bridal shower?
12. Can you use a potholder with a pan?
13. Do you die from getting poison ivy?
14. Can you have two first cousins?
15. Can you have a square meal on a round plate?
16. Can you wear a nightgown during the day?
17. Can a person take a catnap?
18. Can a human being get goose bumps?
19. Is a young bear a cub scout?
20. Can you be color-blind and still be able to see?

Directions: Answer the questions with yes or no.

1. Is Vincent Van Gogh known for being an artist?
2. Is Ed Sullivan known for being a politician?
3. Is Donald Trump known for being a judge?
4. Is George Clooney known for being an actor?
5. Is Ernest Hemingway known for being a writer?
6. Is Barbara Walters known for being a tennis player?
7. Is Cleopatra known for being a pop singer?
8. Is Fred Astaire known for being a dancer?
9. Is Jimmy Carter known for being a country singer?
10. Is Muhammed Ali known for being a boxer?
11. Is Sandra Day O'Connor known for being a news reporter?
12. Is Michael Jordan known for being a basketball player?
13. Is Johnny Carson known for being a president?
14. Is Kevin Costner known for being a senator?
15. Is Charles Dickens known for being a writer?
16. Is Oprah Winfrey known for being a fashion model?
17. Is Tony Bennett known for being a singer?
18. Are the Backstreet Boys known for being a comedy team?
19. Is Ellen Degeneres known for being a comedian?
20. Is Hilary Swank known for being an actor?

Human Qualities

Receptive: Yes / No

Directions: Answer the questions with yes or no.

1. Is an organized person usually neat?
2. Would a frugal person spend frivolously?
3. Would a nostalgic person enjoy old photos?
4. Would a generous person be likely to share?
5. Is a liar someone you would trust?
6. Is a hypochondriac a happy, healthy person?
7. Is a paranoid person usually suspicious?
8. Would a timid person be a loudmouth?
9. Is a hero a good role model?
10. Would a bully be sensitive?
11. Would it be hard to convince a skeptic of a new idea?
12. Would an acquaintance be your best friend?
13. Does a conservative person like to take risks?
14. Would you trust a sincere person?
15. Is an atheist likely to be religious?
16. Is a logical person likely to have common sense?
17. Is it enjoyable to be with an obnoxious person?
18. Does an absent-minded person forget easily?
19. Would a considerate person make a good neighbor?
20. Would a tactful person be insulting?

Directions: Answer the questions with yes or no.

1. If it is Sunday, is it a weekend?
2. If a car is out of fuel, will it run?
3. If a lightbulb is burned out, can it be recharged?
4. If weeds are not watered, will they still grow?
5. If a baby is three months old, can it walk?
6. If a restaurant is closed until further notice, can you eat there tomorrow?
7. If you get a flu shot, can you still catch the flu?
8. If a dog is neutered, can it father puppies?
9. If you record a TV show, can you watch it later?
10. If you have a power outage, can you flush a toilet?
11. If you have leftovers, can they be reheated?
12. If a credit card has expired, can you still use it?
13. If the temperature is 82°, will icicles form?
14. If magazines are set on fire, will they burn?
15. If a plastic bag has two small holes in it, will it hold pretzels?
16. If a candy is sugar-free, does it have calories?
17. If a food item is low in fat, can you gain weight by eating it?
18. If a street is one way, can you travel on it?
19. If food is wrapped in foil, can it be heated in a microwave?
20. If a piece of clothing is out of date, can you wear it?

All or Some

Directions: Answer the questions with yes or no.

1. Do all plants need sunlight to grow?
2. Do all stores take personal checks?
3. Do all adults have tonsils?
4. Do all businesses go bankrupt at some time?
5. Does passing a driving test always make you a good driver?
6. Is Thanksgiving always on the same day of the week?
7. Do all states have a sales tax?
8. Do all candles have wicks?
9. Do all plants have roots?
10. Do all restaurants serve carry-out foods?
11. Do all homes have basements / cellars?
12. Do all dictionaries contain words?
13. Are all cartoons funny?
14. Do all ice cream products need to be kept frozen?
15. Are all wine bottles sealed with corks?
16. Can all musical instruments play jazz?
17. Do you need 52 cards in a deck to play all card games?
18. Do all handicapped-parking spaces require a special permit to park in them?
19. Does our hearing always get worse as we grow older?
20. Is cancer always fatal?

Directions: Answer the questions with yes or no.

1. Can a fire alarm go off when there isn't a fire?
2. Can you remove spots on clothing without detergent?
3. Can you use a cash register to balance a checkbook?
4. Can you fry food in margarine?
5. Can you get a rash from something you eat?
6. Can you use a magnet to stick a picture on a mirror?
7. Can a woman using birth control become pregnant?
8. Can a package from California be delivered to New York the same day?
9. Can you put bullets in a squirt gun?
10. Can you watch an uncut, uninterrupted movie in your home?
11. Can a refrigerator be powered by batteries?
12. Can someone who is innocent be kept in jail?
13. Can you cook an egg without breaking its shell?
14. Can you reupholster a wooden rocking chair?
15. Can a U.S. citizen have been born in another country?
16. Can you have your gallbladder removed and still live?
17. Can you pour water in a burlap bag and not have it leak?
18. Can you grow cactus in a greenhouse?
19. Can you cut a lobster shell with a knife and fork?
20. Can you take a photograph and also be in the picture?

Necessity

Receptive: Yes / No

Directions: Answer the questions with yes or no.

1. Do you need a zip code to call long distance?
2. Do you need an umpire at a Little League game?
3. Do you need a satellite dish for a large party?
4. Do you need a towrope to water ski?
5. Do you need a bandage for a nosebleed?
6. Do you need a net to play backgammon?
7. Do you need cards to play Bingo?
8. Do you need earphones to hear a radio broadcast?
9. Do you need a putter in a golf bag?
10. Do you need collateral to get a bank loan?
11. Do you need a gun to shoot baskets?
12. Do you need a knife to cut through mousse?
13. Do you need lungs to breathe?
14. Does a car need a license plate on the front and on the back?
15. Do you need a funnel to pour liquids into small openings?
16. Do you need an antibiotic to cure a cold?
17. Do you need a deposit slip to take money from a bank account?
18. Do you need a facelift to get rid of freckles?
19. Do you need a bow to play a cello?
20. Do you need skis to go snowboarding?

Directions: Answer the questions with yes or no.

1. Could you daydream at night?
2. Do you store celery in a freezer?
3. Is a tennis ball hollow?
4. Do some women swim in three-piece suits?
5. Could you get a rash from eating food?
6. Could you get athlete's foot from a locker room?
7. Is a loan shark a fish?
8. Does thunder produce an electrical charge?
9. Are overhangs and hangovers similar?
10. Can you grow silk flowers?
11. Do you peel lima beans before you eat them?
12. Does a pelican have a big bill?
13. Are the credits run at the beginning of a movie?
14. Can you order merchandise over the Internet?
15. Does an atheist regularly attend religious services?
16. Could you stain wood to protect it?
17. Would you fill a syringe with acid?
18. Could you drink a milkshake through a straw?
19. Do you need a college degree to practice bigamy?
20. Would you set an alarm to take a sleeping pill?

Judgment Calls

Directions: Answer the questions with yes or no.

1. Would you spend time in a barn if you were allergic to hay?
2. Would you call the theater if you were going to be late to a movie?
3. Would you use a pen if you were writing a rough draft?
4. Would you turn the lights on when entering a room?
5. Would you count calories if you were dieting?
6. Would you give a baby safety pins to play with?
7. Would you visit someone who you knew was contagious?
8. Would you use milk to dilute orange juice concentrate?
9. Would you have your mail held at the post office if you were going on vacation?
10. Would you drive on the shoulder if traffic was traveling slowly?
11. Would you dial 911 if you were having trouble breathing?
12. Would you use an air conditioner to cool a patio?
13. Would you leave through a door marked NO EXIT?
14. Would you make reservations to stay overnight in a hospital?
15. Would you feel safe jaywalking if there was no traffic?
16. Would you take a gun on a house-hunting trip?
17. Would you offer a cocktail to a member of AA?
18. Would you take a gift to a funeral?
19. Would you ask to take home your uneaten food from a restaurant?
20. Would you see a fertility specialist if your grass wouldn't grow?

Directions: Answer the questions with yes or no.

1. Is chicken broth thinner than beef stew?
2. Does paper take longer to decompose than plastic?
3. Is denim a sturdier fabric than silk?
4. Is it more painful to give blood than to have your blood pressure taken?
5. Is stainless more expensive than sterling?
6. Is a pigeon more colorful than a peacock?
7. Is plywood thicker than veneer?
8. Does Fort Wayne usually have a higher temperature in February than Fort Lauderdale?
9. Does a lime have more juice than a banana?
10. Does a Sunday paper usually have fewer pages than a Monday paper?
11. Is 7-Up less carbonated than apple juice?
12. Is murder a worse crime than trespassing?
13. Is an antipasto eaten before an entrée?
14. Does a canoe hold more people than a kayak?
15. Is skydiving scarier than scuba diving?
16. Is a hypnotist more interested in your future than a psychic?
17. Does cotton shrink more than polyester?
18. Are you more likely to slip on wet sand than on a wet deck?
19. Does a cat generally have a longer life span than a dog?
20. Does it take more schooling to become an electrician than a pediatrician?

Dimensions

Receptive: Yes / No

Directions: Answer the questions with yes or no.

1. Are your toes longer than your fingers?
2. Is a boxing ring larger than a diamond ring?
3. Is a snail shorter than a snake?
4. Is a peach smaller than a plum?
5. Is a mountain taller than a molehill?
6. Is a furnace larger than a fan?
7. Is a minivan longer than a moving van?
8. Is a suspended sentence shorter than a life sentence?
9. Is a greeting card smaller than a business card?
10. Does a sunflower grow taller than a snapdragon?
11. Is a sheet of toilet paper larger than a sheet of paper towel?
12. Is a tongue depressor longer than a toothpick?
13. Is a weekend shorter than a week?
14. Is a head of cauliflower smaller than a head of garlic?
15. Is a steeple taller than a bell tower?
16. Is a basin larger than a bathtub?
17. Is a tennis court longer than a shuffleboard court?
18. Is a towel shorter than a washcloth?
19. Is a clipboard smaller than a bulletin board?
20. Is a chest of drawers taller than an armoire?

Directions: Answer the questions with yes or no.

1. Do you need a pencil to draw a blank?
2. Do you need a bypass if you have a heart of gold?
3. Is something expensive if it costs an arm and a leg?
4. Are you broke if money is no object?
5. Are you upset if you lose your cool?
6. Would you want a shot in the arm if you were down in the dumps?
7. Would you forgive and forget if you tend to hold grudges?
8. Are you happy to get the ax?
9. Is it efficient to kill two birds with one stone?
10. Do you have lots of time if it's down to the wire?
11. Are you sure of yourself if you are on the fence?
12. Can you get away with murder even if you don't kill someone?
13. Are you likely to be up a creek without a paddle if you plan ahead?
14. Can a man get a pink slip?
15. Is it hard to take it easy?
16. Would you make a long story short by getting to the bottom line?
17. Do you thank your lucky stars for a windfall?
18. Do you turn thumbs down on something you want?
19. Do you need to lose something in order to get it all together?
20. Are you listening if something goes in one ear and out the other?

Emotions

Receptive: Yes / No

Directions: Answer the questions with yes or no.

1. Are you bored if a lecture is motivating?
2. Are you lethargic after you eat a very big meal?
3. Are you somber when you are happy?
4. Are you nervous when you are put on the spot?
5. Are you comfortable if you have indigestion?
6. Are you irritated when little things go wrong?
7. Are you envious if someone shows you his/her new bruises?
8. Are you suspicious if you are paranoid?
9. Are you innocent if your conscience is bothering you?
10. Are you hurt if you trust a friend who lets you down?
11. Are you delighted when you are in the dumps?
12. Are you proud when someone pays you a compliment?
13. Are you eager if you are ambivalent?
14. Are you fickle if you take whatever is given to you?
15. Are you excited to do a mediocre job?
16. Are you wary if you hear about a deal that sounds too good to be true?
17. Are you confident if you are out of your element?
18. Are you relieved when a stressful time is over?
19. Are you elated if you are overlooked for a promotion?
20. Are you resentful when you are asked your opinion?

Directions: Answer the questions with yes or no.

1. Does an elevator hold more people than a bus?
2. Would a quart of paint cover an entire garage?
3. Is a movie that lasts three hours considered long?
4. Is 18 years a long time for a dog to live?
5. Does it usually take longer than an hour to walk a mile?
6. Is an acre larger than the size of your yard?
7. Can you drive from Boston to Miami in one day?
8. Does it take you longer than a half hour to eat breakfast?
9. Can 10 keychains fit in a shoe box?
10. Does it usually take about 10 minutes to drive 10 miles?
11. Would you be pleased to make 9 percent on an investment?
12. Does it take longer to make a hamburger than a meat loaf?
13. Is five minutes a long time to wait for a traffic light to change?
14. Is your resting pulse a higher number than your age?
15. Would a head of lettuce make enough salad for two people?
16. Could you fit a dozen hard-boiled eggs in a coffee cup?
17. Does it usually take longer than an hour to read a novel?
18. Is a bathroom normally larger than a kitchen?
19. Is a cat weighing 12 pounds considered large?
20. Would a cup of water fill up a teakettle?

Two Variables

Receptive: Yes / No

Directions: Answer the questions with yes or no.

1. Can a food be both cold and spicy?
2. Can today be both warmer and cooler than yesterday?
3. Can you be exhausted and alert at the same time?
4. Can I be in debt and also have money in my pocket?
5. Can you be both younger and taller than I am?
6. Can you take a shower and a bath at the same time?
7. Can you be angry with someone and still love the person?
8. Can you have a nightmare and a dream in the same night?
9. Can you legally drink alcohol and drive at the same time?
10. Can you be color-blind and still see?
11. Can you practice driving and parking at a driving range?
12. Can you receive a bill and a check on the same day?
13. Can you be both an aunt and an uncle?
14. Can a movie be both sad and funny?
15. Can you see your shadow during the day and at night?
16. Can you be crying and happy at the same time?
17. Can an animal be both wild and tame at the same time?
18. Can a product be expensive and still be a bargain?
19. Can a woman have both twins and triplets?
20. Can a man be bald and still grow facial hair?

Three Variables

Directions: Answer the questions with yes or no.

1. Are cardinals and hawks both birds?
2. Are Mercury and Lincoln both planets?
3. Are peas and squash both vegetables?
4. Are the Rockies and Smokies both mountains?
5. Are baseball and hunting both team sports?
6. Are tubas and drums both fabrics?
7. Are wasps and beetles both insects?
8. Are daisies and pansies both trees?
9. Are skyscrapers and hotels both buildings?
10. Are wrenches and pliers both tools?
11. Are loafers and slippers both furniture?
12. Are Canada and Austria both countries?
13. Are sirloin and tenderloin both seafood?
14. Are Scrabble and Monopoly both games?
15. Are Dell and Gateway both colleges?
16. Are Kristin and Justin both first names?
17. Are bottles and windows both made of metal?
18. Are *Time* and *Newsweek* both magazines?
19. Are a rabbit's foot and a black cat both considered lucky?
20. Are French and German both languages?

Complex Vocabulary

Receptive: Yes / No

Directions: Answer the questions with yes or no.

1. If a warranty expired, would it be valid?
2. If you were anorexic, would you be obese?
3. If a baby were feverish, would you put it in an incubator?
4. If you were hyperventilating, would you be apprehensive?
5. If you were nauseous, would you be contagious?
6. If you woke up shivering, would you use an afghan?
7. If you needed a transplant, would you see a surgeon?
8. If water were purified, would it be contaminated?
9. If you were a recluse, would you crave solitary confinement?
10. If you were cremated, would you be embalmed?
11. If you were blackmailed, would you be charged with conspiracy?
12. If a family were estranged, would they be reunited?
13. If you were Orthodox, would you keep kosher?
14. If you were incontinent, would you need to have dialysis?
15. Would a unanimous vote result in a landslide election?
16. Would a slalom race take place on a bobsled course?
17. Would you improvise an impromptu talk?
18. Would a heathen honor the Sabbath?
19. Would a clearance sale reduce inventory?
20. Would you arbitrate a compromise?

Directions: Answer the questions with yes or no.

1. Can you wear a sock on either foot? Can you wear a shoe on either foot?
2. Can you eat using one hand? Can you eat using both hands?
3. Do you read a page from right to left? Do you read a page from left to right?
4. Can you play soccer with a broken arm? Can you play soccer with a broken leg?
5. Can a hen lay golden eggs? Can a hen lay brown eggs?
6. Can you weigh less than you did five years ago? Can you weigh more than you did five years ago?
7. Can you eat with a paper plate? Can you eat with a paper fork?
8. Can you get money by working for it? Can you get money without working for it?
9. Can you sleep lying down? Can you sleep sitting up?
10. Can you eat dark chocolate? Can you eat white chocolate?
11. Can a woman get pregnant? Can a man get pregnant?
12. Do you eat raw tomatoes? Do you eat cooked tomatoes?
13. Can you travel by car to the Bahamas? Can you travel by ship to the Bahamas?
14. Can you have nine dollars in bills? Can you have nine dollars in coins?
15. Do you shave the hair on your legs? Do you shave the hair on your face?
16. Can you write with your left hand? Can you write with your right hand?
17. Can you walk on water? Can you swim in water?
18. Can you live without a heart? Can you live without a brain?
19. Can you go down a floor in an escalator? Can you go up a floor in an elevator?
20. Do you need a license to drive a car? Do you need a license to drive a bicycle?

Multiple Variables

Receptive: Yes / No

Directions: Answer the questions with yes or no.

1. Are oysters and octopuses both saltwater shellfish?
2. Are beets and carrots both root vegetables?
3. Are pepperoni and minestrone both spicy Italian foods?
4. Are luge and speed skating both winter Olympic events?
5. Do songs and poems both contain verses and a chorus?
6. Are shoes and belts sized by both length and width?
7. Are rams and moose both animals with horns?
8. Are corsets and Corvettes both antique clothing?
9. Are honey and wet tar both soft and sticky?
10. Are andirons and bellows both equipment for gas and log fireplaces?
11. Are bagels and oatmeal both cold breakfast foods?
12. Are Maalox and Tums both medicines for an upset stomach?
13. Are Anchorage and Antarctica both cold countries?
14. Are flutes and tubas both musical instruments you blow?
15. Are cabbage and lettuce both green and round?
16. Are yoga and jogging both aerobic exercises?
17. Are Chicago and Boston both musical plays and movies?
18. Are pines and palms both trees that lose their leaves in winter?
19. Are Barbra Streisand and Jennifer Lopez singers who also make movies?
20. Are orange and peach both fruit and colors?

Directions: Keep in mind the object referred to and answer the questions with yes or no.

1. Think about an oil painting.
   Could it increase in value? Could it burn? Could it be framed? Could it be erased?

2. Think about a computer.
   Could it help you figure your taxes? Could it make dinner? Could it break down? Could you play chess with it?

3. Think about a limousine.
   Is it a means of transportation? Is it smaller than a Thunderbird? Is it used to go camping? Can it hold more than four people?

4. Think about closets.
   Can they be used for storage? Can they have shelves? Can you buy them? Can one be used as a bedroom?

5. Think about a flashlight.
   Is it too heavy to hold? Does it run on electricity? Can it be used indoors and outdoors? Is it more likely to be used in the day than at night?

6. Think about a pair of gloves.
   Could they be made of leather? Could they come in different colors and sizes? Could they be washed? Could you buy only one?

7. Think about a DVD player.
   Do you need a computer to use it? Can you take photos with it? Can you show movies with it? Can it run on batteries?

8. Think about a dictionary.
   Can it have pictures in it? Can it be in a foreign language? Do all dictionaries define the same words? Can it be on disk?

9. Think about a sweater.
   Does it come in different sizes and colors? Is it worn over a coat? Can it stretch? Can it have a collar?

10. Think of a piano.
    Does it have keys? Can it be electric? Can anyone learn to play? Can it be played with one hand?

11. Think about a suit.
    Do all suits have a vest? Can it range in price? Can a woman's suit have a skirt? Are all suits washable?

12. Think about a beaver.
    Can it swim? Does it have a short tail? Does it like water? Does it have sharp teeth?

13. Think about a watermelon.
    Would you eat it hot? Do you eat the seeds? Do you eat the skin? Is it a vegetable?

14. Think about athletic shoes.
    Do they come in colors? Are they made out of different materials? Do they have leather soles? Do you polish them?

15. Think about fleas.
    Can they live anywhere? Can you set traps to remove them? Do they eat other bugs? Can they bite humans?

16. Think about a blow-dryer for your hair.
    Would you keep it in a bedroom? Can it blow hot or cool? Do you need training to use it? Is it portable?

17. Think about a rose.
    Are roses houseplants? Do they come in different colors? Do all roses have long stems? Are they grown from a bulb?

18. Think about the president of the United States.
    Could a woman have the job? Could a president serve for 12 years? Is it necessary to be a senator before running for president? Does the president have to live in the White House?

19. Think about feathers.
    Do animals and birds have them? Can they be man-made? Can they be put back on after they are shed? Are they used for decoration?

20. Think about milk.
    Can it be stored anywhere? Can it be drunk hot or cold? Can people be allergic to it? Can it come from animals other than cows?

MULTIPLE CHOICE

55 Orientation ....*Are you a man or a woman?*

56 Verb Choices..............................*Do you fry or boil water?*

57 Categories ....*Is a spy a person or an animal?*

58 Characteristics............................*Does lard or turpentine remove paint?*

59 Facts ....*Do skirts or slacks have inseams?*

60 Similar Meanings........................*Does a hitch or a jack attach to a trailer?*

61 Similar Sounding Words............*Would it be freezing or sneezing cold outside?*

62 Locations...................................*Would you find animation in a cartoon or a comic strip?*

63 Similarities................................*Does a chimp or a cheetah look more like a cat?*

64 Jobs ....*Does a referee or an emcee host a show?*

65 Celebrities ....*Is Matt Laurer or Matt Damon an actor?*

66 Historical Names ....*Was Julius Caesar a philosopher or an emperor?*

67 Geography.................................*Are the Cayman Islands in the Mediterranean or the Caribbean Sea?*

68 Brand Recognition.....................*Ex-Lax and Windex. Name the glass cleaner.*

69 Better Idea.................................*Which is a better idea? To write a check with a pen or a pencil*

70 Visualize ....*Is the green traffic light above or below the yellow one?*

71 Basic Comparisons ....*What is strong? paper or steel*

72 Features.....................................*What has strings? flute or harp*

73 Compound Words ....*Which one do you chew? bubblegum or bubble bath*

74 Comparisons ....*Which is longer? semester or year*

75 Order of Events..........................*Do you wax a floor before or after you wash it?*

76 First and Last ....*Which is first? ashes or fire*

77 Three Choices.............................*Which is a shellfish? salmon shrimp trout*

78 Superlatives................................*Which is the fastest? cheetah bicycle digestion*

79 Unnecessary Items......................*Which is not necessary to take care of a cut? antiseptic water aspirin*

80 Recognize Parts ....*Which two words are parts of a cat? whiskers tail copper beak*

81 Complex Questions.....................*Is it easier or harder to walk uphill than downhill?*

MULTIPLE CHOICE

Directions: Choose the correct answer from the choices.

1. Are you a man or a woman?
2. Is it the morning or the afternoon?
3. Is it a weekday or the weekend?
4. Is the weather warm or cool?
5. Are you wearing street clothes or night clothes?
6. Are you lying down or sitting up?
7. Do you live alone or with someone?
8. Are you usually right- or left-handed?
9. Are you shorter or taller than your father?
10. Is your hair naturally straight or curly?
11. (city) Do you live in _________ or _________ ?
12. (state) Do you live in _________ or _________ ?
13. Are you at home or in an office?
14. Are you wearing pants or a skirt?
15. Do you use a wheelchair or a cane?
16. Are you under 50 or over 50 years old?
17. Do you prefer to drink soft drinks or water?
18. Do you have dark, light, or gray hair?
19. Have you ever had a dog, a cat, or a bird?
20. Are you in school, working, or retired?

Verb Choices

Directions: Choose the correct answer from the choices.

1. Do you fry or boil water?
2. Do you brush or comb your teeth?
3. Do you burn or plant a garden?
4. Do you shovel or cut dirt?
5. Do you saw or hammer tree limbs?
6. Do you question or answer a ringing phone?
7. Do you chew or suck gum?
8. Do you knit or sew yarn?
9. Do you see or hear a noise?
10. Do you sing or dance a lullaby?
11. Do you sleep or swim in a pool?
12. Do you throw or catch a cold?
13. Do you watch or clean a soap opera?
14. Do you eat or wear moccasins?
15. Do you push or carry a grocery cart?
16. Do you mow or plow snow?
17. Do you stand or sit on a throne?
18. Do you cut or curl your fingernails?
19. Do you smash or slice cheese?
20. Do you read or write a map?

Directions: Choose the correct answer from the choices.

1. Is a spy a person or an animal?
2. Is a Reuben a salad or a sandwich?
3. Is W a number or a letter?
4. Is Naples a city or a state?
5. Is Disneyland a museum or a theme park?
6. Is cabbage a fruit or a vegetable?
7. Is beige a color or clothing?
8. Are candles decoration or food?
9. Is Cuba an ocean or an island?
10. Is a pistol a gun or a flower?
11. Is a dove an insect or a bird?
12. Is a black widow a spider or a snake?
13. Is penicillin candy or medicine?
14. Is a waltz a dance or a musical instrument?
15. Is a pecan a drink or a nut?
16. Is a bull a male or a female?
17. Is Colgate a deodorant or a toothpaste?
18. Is bamboo pottery or wood?
19. Is moss found in a forest or a desert?
20. Is autumn a season or a month?

Characteristics

Receptive: Multiple Choice

Directions: Choose the correct answer from the choices.

1. Does lard or turpentine remove paint?
2. Do boats or tractors use anchors?
3. Do pine trees or oak trees grow acorns?
4. Do prunes or bananas have pits?
5. Do beavers or porcupines have quills?
6. Does sugar or sand dissolve in hot water?
7. Do trays or cabinets have drawers?
8. Does a tiger or a lion have a mane?
9. Does a sleeping bag or a mattress roll up?
10. Do pretzels or grapes grow on vines?
11. Does blood or water run through your veins?
12. Do oceans or rivers have salt water?
13. Does a truck or a bus have an aisle?
14. Does a sliding door or a staircase have a railing?
15. Do bones or muscles get sprained?
16. Does a corkscrew or a screwdriver open a bottle of wine?
17. Does a helicopter or a car have propellers?
18. Do logs or candles have wicks?
19. Does a library or a café have books?
20. Does an Eskimo pie or a potpie have a crust?

Directions: Choose the correct answer from the choices.

1. Do skirts or slacks have inseams?
2. Does wood or metal conduct electricity?
3. Is perfume or cologne generally more expensive?
4. Is mascara or eyeliner used on eyelashes?
5. Would you shop or eat at a banquet?
6. Can you see through transparent or opaque material?
7. Does an astronaut or an astrologer travel into space?
8. Is a mermaid real or imaginary?
9. Would a child carry a backpack or a six-pack to school?
10. Are vitamins or aspirin prescribed for pain?
11. Would a defendant appeal a conviction or an acquittal?
12. Does a cat purr or hiss if it is upset?
13. Would you use dough for a piecrust or a pie filling?
14. Is chrome silver or gold in color?
15. Are there more palm trees growing in Alaska or Arizona?
16. Does a piece of wood or steel float?
17. Would a man be a widow or a widower?
18. Do closets have rods or reels?
19. Does a book or a play have a script?
20. Do you use an emery board or cardboard to file your nails?

Similar Meanings

Receptive: Multiple Choice

Directions: Choose the correct answer from the choices.

1. Does a hitch or a jack attach to a trailer?
2. Does a dead bolt or a chain lock provide more security?
3. Are sunglasses or goggles used underwater?
4. Does ash or sawdust remain after a fire?
5. Does a thermometer or a thermostat regulate the temperature in a room?
6. Does an index or a table of contents come at the end of a book?
7. Does a Jacuzzi or a sauna use dry heat?
8. Is venom or saliva poisonous?
9. Is a person's silhouette or a shadow able to be framed?
10. Does a rerun or a replay happen instantly?
11. Do earplugs or earmuffs keep ears warm?
12. Do blinds or shutters roll up?
13. Does a koala bear or a polar bear eat fish?
14. If you don't have health insurance, can you apply for Medicaid or medication?
15. Does cocoa or coffee contain caffeine?
16. Do you put frosting on a cupcake or a biscuit?
17. Does a secretary or a treasurer handle the money?
18. Are most states divided into counties or countries?
19. Do the kidneys or the liver aid in digestion?
20. Does a sorority or a fraternity have women members?

Directions: Choose the correct answer from the choices.

1. Would it be freezing or sneezing cold outside?
2. Would you sweep rust or dust under a rug?
3. Would you throw old rags or hags into a trash can?
4. Would a hog or a frog hop onto a rock?
5. Would a jeep or a creep need a yearly tune-up?
6. Would you be congratulated on being engaged or enraged?
7. Does ham or lamb come from pigs?
8. Would you have a star or a scar after getting stitches?
9. Are pimples or dimples more desirable on the face?
10. Would you take antibiotics or antifreeze if you had the flu?
11. Would you scratch or patch a hole in a wall?
12. Would you put a coaster or a canister under a glass?
13. Would you want to be with someone who was devoted or devious?
14. Would you prefer a receiver or a retriever for a pet?
15. Would a shirt or a skirt have a button-down collar?
16. Would you use a hatchet or a ratchet to loosen a bolt?
17. Would you spank or thank a child for misbehaving?
18. Would you cash or slash a check made out to you?
19. Would someone wear a Rolodex or a Rolex on the wrist?
20. Would you be more likely to get a message or a massage during a business meeting?

Locations

Receptive: Multiple Choice

Directions: Choose the correct answer from the choices.

1. Would you find animation in a cartoon or a comic strip?
2. Would you sail a boat in a harbor or a dock?
3. Would you find an editorial in a book or a newspaper?
4. Would you plan a shopping trip to a mall or a hall?
5. Would a sewer line be installed above or below ground?
6. Would you cook in a tidal wave or a microwave?
7. Would you find a turnstile at a subway station or a stationery store?
8. Would you put a horse in a padlock or a paddock?
9. Would you go to an auditorium for a lecture or a hearing test?
10. Would you buy soft drinks or beer in a keg?
11. Would floss or moss be kept in a medicine cabinet?
12. Would a mallet or a hatchet be part of a croquet set?
13. Would you sit in a balcony or a basement at a concert hall?
14. Would you go to a model home or an open house for a party?
15. Is a microphone or a microscope used in a science lab?
16. Would you buy a corsage or a corset at a florist?
17. Would you find Post-It Notes or posters on a desk?
18. Would you go to a nursery or a bakery to purchase strudel?
19. Would bats or shovels be in a dugout?
20. Would you put dirty or clean clothes in a garment bag?

Directions: Choose the correct answer from the choices.

1. Does a chimp or a cheetah look more like a cat?
2. Does a refrigerator or a card table cost about the same as a sofa?
3. Is a briefcase or a piano bench about as long as a yardstick?
4. Is a tree or a bush about as tall as a two-story house?
5. Is a motorcycle or a truck about the size of a bus?
6. Is a sheep or a raccoon about the same size as a golden retriever?
7. Is a lamp or a night-light about as bright as a votive candle?
8. Does meatloaf or lasagna taste more like hamburger?
9. Is the shape of a bagel or a brownie about the same as a doughnut?
10. Is a beach or a couch about as soft as a bed?
11. Is a can of Coke or a bottle of wine about the same height as a carton of milk?
12. Does cabbage or celery look more like lettuce?
13. Is changing a lightbulb or changing jobs about as complicated as changing a baby?
14. Was the assassination of Kennedy or the resignation of Nixon about the same time as Watergate?
15. Is sorbet or pudding about as cold as ice cream?
16. Does Sacramento or Chicago get about as cold as Orlando?
17. Is a soccer ball or a tennis ball about the same size as a basketball?
18. Does a deer or a rabbit run at about the same speed as a horse?
19. Is a credit card or a dollar bill about the same size as a check?
20. Is an ant or a cockroach about the same size as a mosquito?

Jobs

Directions: Choose the correct answer from the choices.

1. Does a referee or an emcee host a show?
2. Does an electrician or a surgeon perform surgery?
3. Does a police officer or a social worker use handcuffs?
4. Does a chef or a hockey player use a face mask?
5. Does a jeweler or a gold digger sell gold?
6. Does a jockey or a carpenter use a sawhorse?
7. Does a realtor or a writer sell homes?
8. Does a waiter or a grocer buy and sell food?
9. Does a construction worker or a weather forecaster use a hard hat?
10. Does a chauffeur or a pilot drive people?
11. Does a pedestrian or a pediatrician treat children?
12. Does a comedian or a senator pass laws?
13. Does a plumber or an architect repair pipes?
14. Does a governor or a president lead the country?
15. Does a criminal or a lawyer break the law?
16. Does a psychologist or a pianist play music?
17. Does a football player or a swimmer wear a helmet?
18. Does a dentist or a therapist use a drill?
19. Does a student or a professor teach classes?
20. Does a firefighter or a welder use an oxygen mask?

Directions: Choose the correct answer from the choices.

1. Is Matt Laurer or Matt Damon an actor?
2. Is Billy Joel or Billy Crystal a singer?
3. Is Dick Clark or Clark Kent also Superman?
4. Does Larry King or Stephen King write novels?
5. Is Garth Brooks or Brooke Shields a country singer?
6. Did Ray Romano or Jay Leno take Johnny Carson's place?
7. Is Beyonce or Emeril a chef?
8. Is George Clooney or George Carlin an actor?
9. Is Howard Dean or Howard Stern a radio personality?
10. Is Al Pacino or Al Roker a weatherman?
11. Is Robin Williams or William Macy a comedian?
12. Does Martha Stewart or Jon Stewart host a news show?
13. Is Jesse Jackson or Michael Jackson a reverend?
14. Is Kevin Kline or Calvin Klein a fashion designer?
15. Is Steve Martin or Martin Sheen known for dramatic acting?
16. Is Gene Kelly or Grace Kelly known for dancing?
17. Is Jamie Lee Curtis related to Spike Lee or Tony Curtis?
18. Does David Letterman or David Chappelle have a late-night talk show?
19. Is Leonardo da Vinci or Leonardo DiCaprio an artist?
20. Is Sharon Stone or Stone Philips a newscaster?

Historical Names

Receptive: Multiple Choice

Directions: Choose the correct answer from the choices.

1. Was Julius Caesar a philosopher or an emperor?
2. Was Lou Gehrig a golfer or a baseball player?
3. Did Frank Lloyd Wright design houses or paint landscapes?
4. Did Charles Darwin develop the theory of relativity or of evolution?
5. Did Sigmund Freud write about psychology or science fiction?
6. Did Ferdinand Marcos rule Spain or the Philippines?
7. Was Indira Gandhi an East Indian or an American Indian?
8. Was Marco Polo an Olympic champion or an explorer?
9. Was Thomas Edison an inventor or a playwright?
10. Was Dr. Martin Luther King a physician or a minister?
11. Was Jesse James or James Madison a western outlaw?
12. Was Benjamin Franklin or Franklin Roosevelt an inventor?
13. Did Thomas Jefferson or Abraham Lincoln abolish slavery?
14. Did Isaac Newton or Wayne Newton discover the laws of gravity?
15. Was Robert Kennedy or John Kennedy an American president?
16. Was Daniel Boone or Jack Daniels an explorer?
17. Was Norman Rockwell or Norman Schwarzkopf a painter?
18. Was Michelangelo or Shakespeare a writer?
19. Was Stalin or Socrates a Greek philosopher?
20. Was Neil Armstrong or J. Paul Getty the first man on the moon?

Directions: Choose the correct answer from the choices.

1. Are the Cayman Islands in the Mediterranean or the Caribbean Sea?
2. Is Pearl Harbor in the Atlantic or the Pacific Ocean?
3. Is New England in Britain or America?
4. Are the Great Lakes in North or Central America?
5. Is Norway or Holland also known as the Netherlands?
6. Is San Diego or San Francisco farther north?
7. Is Australia or Austria a continent?
8. Does the Panama or the Suez Canal connect the Atlantic and Pacific Oceans?
9. Is Quebec in France or Canada?
10. Is Brazil or Belgium in South America?
11. Is Alaska or Hawaii an island?
12. Are the Rockies or the Smokies west of the Mississippi River?
13. Would you go on a safari in Kenya or China?
14. Is Cape Cod in Minnesota or Massachusetts?
15. Is Niagara Falls on the border of the United States and Mexico or Canada?
16. Is Red Square in Russia or China?
17. Is Key West on the Atlantic or the Pacific Ocean?
18. Was New York or New Orleans hit hardest by Hurricane Katrina?
19. Are the Alps in Europe or the United States?
20. Is Iraq closer to Japan or Afghanistan?

Brand Recognition

Directions: Choose the correct answer from the choices.

1. Ex-Lax and Windex. Name the glass cleaner.
2. Ivory and Ebony. Name the soap.
3. Frito and Oreo. Name the cookie.
4. Preparation H and Special K. Name the cereal.
5. Avis and Avon. Name the rental agency.
6. Land O'Lakes and Ocean Spray. Name the juice.
7. Checkers and Dominos. Name the pizza brand.
8. Maidenform or Rubbermaid. Name the underwear.
9. Dry Idea and Wet Wipes. Name the deodorant.
10. Pepperidge Farm and State Farm. Name the insurance company.
11. Dr. Pepper and Dr. Scholl's. Name the soft drink.
12. Uncle Ben and Bengay. Name the ointment.
13. Healthy Choice and Taster's Choice. Name the frozen meal.
14. Cheerios and Cheer. Name the detergent.
15. Cannon and Dannon. Name the towels.
16. Secret and Shout. Name the stain remover.
17. Hefty and Brawny. Name the paper towels.
18. Saturn and Mars. Name the car.
19. Fruit of the Loom and Froot Loops. Name the food.
20. Miracle Whip and Miracle-Gro. Name the dressing.

Directions: Choose the correct answer from the choices.

Which is a better idea . . .

1. to write a check with a pen or a pencil
2. to put a heating pad or an ice pack on a swollen bruise
3. to put too much or not enough postage on a letter
4. to argue with a mugger or give him what he wants
5. to stop at or go through a yellow traffic light
6. to wash windows on a sunny or a rainy day
7. to get rid of grease by pouring it down a sink or into a can
8. to overcook or undercook vegetables
9. to recycle newspapers or throw them out
10. to have a verbal or a written agreement
11. to dial 911 or call a friend in an emergency
12. to exercise twice a week or twice a month
13. to slice food toward you or away from you
14. to pay your bills monthly or yearly
15. to walk in the dark or turn on a light
16. to buy stock when the price is high or low
17. to return a purchase or throw it out
18. to bet money or invest it
19. to take small or large bites of food
20. to refrigerate leftovers or eat them right away

Visualize

Receptive: Multiple Choice

Directions: Choose the correct answer from the choices.

1. Is the green traffic light above or below the yellow one?
2. Are the buttonholes on your coat on the right or on the left side as you look down?
3. As you look at a faucet, is the hot spigot on the right or the left?
4. Which is the longer hand on a clock—the minute or the hour hand?
5. Do you live on the north, south, east, or west side of the street?
6. When you clap, do you put your right hand in your left or vice versa?
7. Is the coin slot on most vending machines on the right or the left?
8. Are your eyes the same or a different color from your father's?
9. When a light switch is in the up position, is it on or off?
10. Does a stop sign have seven or eight sides?
11. Is Washington or Lincoln on a dollar bill?
12. Do you sleep on the right, left, or middle of a bed?
13. Is a railroad crossing sign or a yield sign in the shape of a triangle?
14. Are the handles on your kitchen cabinets on the side or on the bottom?
15. Is the postmark on the top left or right of an envelope?
16. Does a telephone number have eight or 11 digits?
17. Do you turn on your bath below or above where the water comes out?
18. Does a boxer have a short or a long tail?
19. Are the turn signals on the right or the left of the steering column of a car?
20. When you unscrew a jar lid, do you turn it clockwise or counterclockwise?

Directions: Choose the correct answer from the choices.

1. What is strong? paper or steel
2. What floats? beach ball or bowling ball
3. What can you see through? coal or crystal
4. What is sweet? fudge or fries
5. What is dangerous? rock climbing or rock collecting
6. What holds more? pocket or duffle bag
7. What is spicy? Tabasco sauce or apple juice
8. What is noisy? breathing or snoring
9. What is round? box or ball
10. What stings? wasp or butterfly
11. What is soft? bed or board
12. What is chewy? chocolate or caramel
13. What is destructive? tornado or eclipse
14. What smells sweet? garlic or cinnamon
15. What is crunchy? potato chips or potato pancakes
16. What is tame? parrot or parakeet
17. What is deep? gorge or shore
18. What is man-made? vinyl or clay
19. What burns? log or brick
20. What evaporates? oil or water

Features

Directions: Choose the correct answer from the choices.

1. What has strings? flute or harp
2. What is transparent? tote bag or Ziploc bag
3. What ties only around the neck? bib or apron
4. What has an expiration date? paper towels or cookies
5. What has seeds? cantaloupe or cherry
6. What can tarnish? gold or silver
7. What has coils? electric stove or gas stove
8. What is done standing up? bath or shower
9. What has green skin? potato or cucumber
10. What has bubbles? champagne or cocoa
11. What is the female? niece or nephew
12. What is open to everyone? public or private
13. What is held in one hand? rifle or revolver
14. What pumps blood? the lungs or heart
15. What has spots? leopard or tiger
16. What is a legal resident? citizen or alien
17. What gives you money? bill or refund
18. What is alive? mannequin or model
19. What operates below ground level? subway or trolley
20. What occurs in cold weather? tornado or blizzard

Directions: Choose the correct answer from the choices.

1. Which one do you chew? bubblegum or bubble bath
2. Which one wipes up spills? sandpaper or paper towels
3. Which one is sweet? cheeseburger or cheesecake
4. Which one do you wear? turtleneck or redneck
5. Which one requires a pencil? jigsaw puzzle or crossword puzzle
6. Which one is a college degree? master of ceremonies or master of arts
7. Which one is candy? lima beans or jelly beans
8. Which one is a good thing? bull's eye or black eye
9. Which one is part of a car? fan belt or leather belt
10. Which one would you get a ticket for? double-dating or double-parking
11. Which one could you ride in? Ferris wheel or roulette wheel
12. Which one could you buy? German shepherd or German measles
13. Which one can earn you money? birth certificate or certificate of deposit
14. Which one is worn in water? bathing suit or three-piece suit
15. Which one starts a gas burner? pilot light or floodlight
16. Which one can you use at a future date? check mark or rain check
17. Which one can you bet on? horse race or rat race
18. Which one keeps hair in place? bobby pins or safety pins
19. Which one has a hole in the middle? peanut or doughnut
20. Which one has a sink? restroom or coatroom

Comparisons

Directions: Choose the correct answer from the choices.

1. Which is longer? semester or year
2. Which is brighter? lightning or night-light
3. Which is stronger? wire or string
4. Which is heavier? platter or sponge
5. Which lasts longer? muscle cramp or pulled muscle
6. Which is faster? space shuttle or jet
7. Which happens more often? quarterly or every other month
8. Which spoils faster? coffee cream or coffee ice cream
9. Which takes more skill? playing darts or playing hockey
10. Which cooks the longest? chili or rice
11. Which is more nutritious? bowl of pudding or bowl of salad
12. Which goes higher? hot-air balloon or helium balloon
13. Which provides more heat? kerosene heater or gas furnace
14. Which is more controversial? abortion or adoption
15. Which has more squares? tic-tac-toe grid or bingo card
16. Which is statistically safer? flying in a plane or riding in a car
17. Which holds more? water bottle or water heater
18. Which breaks more easily? plastic or ceramic
19. Which is easier to tear? masking tape or duct tape
20. Which is younger? lamb or sheep

Directions: Choose the correct answer from the choices.

1. Do you wax a floor before or after you wash it?
2. Do you have a wedding before or after a honeymoon?
3. Do you file an insurance claim before or after an accident?
4. Do you learn to swim before or after you learn to water-ski?
5. Is the accused sentenced before or after a verdict?
6. When packing a grocery bag, do you put canned goods in before or after the fresh produce?
7. Do you sterilize a needle before or after you give a shot?
8. Do you peel a hard-boiled egg before or after you cook it?
9. Do you get a flu shot before or after you get the flu?
10. Do you iron a shirt before or after you wash it?
11. Do you put clothes in a dryer before or after you put them in a washer?
12. Do you peel an onion before or after you chop it?
13. Was the assassination of President Kennedy before or after the shooting of President Reagan?
14. Do you serve soup before or after the main course?
15. Do you sign a credit slip before or after it is filled out?
16. Do you put oil in an engine before or after it has run out?
17. Do you put lotion on your skin before or after you shower?
18. Do you celebrate your birthday before or after Labor Day?
19. Do you mash potatoes before or after cooking them?
20. Do you leave a message before or after you hear the beep?

First and Last

Directions: Choose the correct answer from the choices.

1. Which is first? ashes or fire
2. Which is first? introduction or conclusion
3. Which is first? blanket or bedspread
4. Which is first? sunset or sunrise
5. Which is first? surgery or recovery
6. Which is first? Friday or Tuesday
7. Which is first? wash or iron
8. Which is first? adulthood or childhood
9. Which is first? record player or tape recorder
10. Which is first? arrest or trial
11. Which is last? delivery or order
12. Which is last? bread or dough
13. Which is last? salad or dessert
14. Which is last? death or birth
15. Which is last? hiring or firing
16. Which is last? frog or tadpole
17. Which is last? July or February
18. Which is last? marriage or divorce
19. Which is last? morning or afternoon
20. Which is last? swallowing or chewing

Directions: Choose the correct answer from the choices.

1. Which is a shellfish? salmon shrimp trout
2. Which is silver in color? pewter bronze copper
3. Which has stripes down its back? squirrel chipmunk rabbit
4. Which is a dessert? quiche pâté mousse
5. Which is a musical instrument? forceps harmonica odometer
6. Which has a moral? joke story fable
7. Which must happen? wish command prediction
8. Which lands on water? Jet Ski hydroplane helicopter
9. Which is man-made? marble granite formica
10. Which contains the most carbohydrates? pasta pork peanuts
11. Which is drunk? ammonia vodka vinegar
12. Which shows stars? aquarium auditorium planetarium
13. Which is a natural phenomenon? Hollywood Redwoods Dollywood
14. Which is the most portable? iPod plasma TV GPS (global positioning system)
15. Which has slats? egg carton wooden crate gift box
16. Which religion is headed by the Pope? Catholicism Judaism Buddhism
17. Which is tame? anteater warthog guinea pig
18. Which probably contains herbs? pancakes soup cereal
19. Which is a race? Kentucky Derby Superbowl Academy Awards
20. Which is used to clean clothing? cleanser detergent scouring pads

Superlatives

Directions: Choose the correct answer from the choices.

1. Which is the fastest? cheetah bicycle digestion
2. Which is the loudest? baby crying speedboat jet landing
3. Which weighs the most? floor lamp bed pillow stapler
4. Which is the thinnest? sandwich wallet ruler
5. Which lasts the longest? sunburn TV commercial chewing-gum flavor
6. Which is the deepest? ice chest well puddle
7. Which is the widest? Monopoly board chair seat doorway
8. Which is the highest? ranch house water tower traffic light
9. Which is the most dangerous? eating raw poultry diving into a pool having a shot
10. Which has the most legs? spider armchair bumblebee
11. Which is the shortest? penguin two-liter bottle suitcase
12. Which stretches the most? rubber band blanket Slinky
13. Which has the most calories? chocolate cake chocolate kiss chocolate milk
14. Which is the longest? bacon strip baseball bat shoelaces
15. Which is the tallest? staircase stilts picket fence
16. Which has the longest legs? pelican swan flamingo
17. Which is the smallest? dust mite atom grain of sand
18. Which bite is the worst? flea turtle scorpion
19. Which is the lightest? down comforter wet blanket bushel of apples
20. Which holds the most? bucket trunk of a car laundry hamper

Directions: Choose the correct answer from the choices.

Which item is not necessary to . . .

1. take care of a cut? antiseptic water aspirin
2. make pancakes? skillet glass batter
3. repair cracks in pavement? hoe trowel mortar
4. fix a rip in a pair of jeans? patch knife needle
5. make lemon meringue pie? pie shell egg whites lemonade
6. go skiing? skis shoulder pads poles
7. make a bed? towel pillow sheet
8. amuse a child? patience toys diapers
9. marry someone? blood test wedding rings marriage license
10. remove a splinter? magnifying glass needle thread
11. balance a checkbook? credit cards bank statements record of checks
12. make a sundae? topping cream ice cream
13. play poker? scorecard cards chips
14. clean a bathtub? sponge paper towels cleanser
15. polish shoes? cloth polish water
16. clean a pan with baked-on food? scouring pad vinegar hot water
17. trim your own hair? razor blade mirror scissors
18. cook a turkey? roasting pan meat thermometer giblets
19. play a game of pool? billiards table cue stick set of clubs
20. go on the Internet? computer printer network connection

Recognize Parts

Receptive: Multiple Choice

Directions: Choose the correct answers from the choices.

Which two words are . . .

1. parts of a cat? whiskers tail copper beak
2. parts of a salad? cream lettuce stock carrot
3. parts of a book? spoons chapters pages music
4. parts of a body? spleen land pancreas string
5. parts of a tree? roots paws arches branches
6. parts of a kitchen? magic stove pavement faucet
7. parts of a car? dashboard turnpike hood shoulder blade
8. parts of a hotel? elevator nursery theater lobby
9. parts of an elephant? fins tusks trunk feathers
10. parts of a foot? meal zipper arch toes
11. parts of a bed? mattress sheets friend cement
12. parts of a toolbox? screws pipes collar wire
13. parts of a camera? nose bucket shutter lens
14. parts of a newspaper? shorts comics headlines shadows
15. parts of an orchestra? tub violent flute clarinet
16. parts of a lamp? bulb sheet lid cord
17. parts of a mouth? glue tongue lips brow
18. parts of a bathroom? toilet sink bat refrigerator
19. parts of an office? computer piano grass desk
20. parts of a watch? heater face band collar

Directions: Choose the correct answer from the choices.

1. Is it easier or harder to walk uphill than downhill?
2. Is it better or worse to take aspirin than to take cocaine?
3. Is it more or less healthy to climb two flights of stairs than to walk four miles?
4. Is it more or less advantageous to read the directions than to just turn on a new appliance?
5. Does it save more or less money to buy food in bulk than to shop as you need items?
6. Is it easier or harder to make a pie than to make spaghetti?
7. Is someone who is old enough for school but not old enough to drive, old enough to read or vote?
8. Does it get darker earlier or later in January than in July?
9. Are there fewer or more illustrations in an atlas than in a dictionary?
10. Is it easier or harder to renew a magazine subscription than a driver's license?
11. In general, is it more or less likely that politicians say what will get them elected rather than what they truly feel?
12. Is it better or worse to lay an extension cord for outside decorations across a sidewalk than across the grass?
13. Is it less or more correct to send the hostess money after a party than a thank-you note?
14. Would you be more or less liable to hurt yourself when jumping rope than bungee jumping?
15. Would it be better or worse to reheat a pizza in the oven than on the stove?
16. Are you less or more liable to use storm windows than screens to keep your house warmer in winter?
17. Are there more or fewer guest rooms in a hotel than in a bed and breakfast?
18. Is it better or worse to drink six beers a day than two?
19. Does it cost more or less to buy a used car than to buy a new car?
20. Is it more or less dangerous to take too many sleeping pills than vitamins?

SENTENCE COMPREHENSION

Directions: Follow the instructions.

1. Show me your palms.
2. Stick out your tongue.
3. Snap your fingers.
4. Make a "thumbs-down" sign.
5. Put your tongue between your teeth.
6. Look over one shoulder.
7. Pretend you are chewing gum.
8. Drop your jaw.
9. Pat your stomach.
10. Hum a tune.
11. Suck in your cheeks.
12. Draw a circle in the air.
13. Cross your fingers.
14. Wrinkle your eyebrows.
15. Pull on your earlobe.
16. Scratch your scalp.
17. Touch the back of your neck.
18. Put your little finger and thumb together.
19. Press your ear to your shoulder.
20. Smile with your mouth closed.

Scanning Directions

Directions: Follow the instructions.

1. Pick up the closest object to you.
2. Point to something behind you.
3. Show me a freckle on your arm.
4. Point to the largest piece of furniture you can see.
5. Point to where you turn on a light.
6. Point to two things that are about the same size.
7. Point to your longest fingernail.
8. Point to two of the same thing.
9. Point to something on the wall.
10. Point to a corner in the ceiling.
11. If you can find a dirty spot, point to it.
12. Point to something that would burn in a fire.
13. Where is the light fixture in the room?
14. Point to something that is plugged in.
15. If there is a phone, point to it.
16. Point to all of the chairs in the room.
17. If you have a scar, show it to me.
18. Where is the doorway?
19. Show which one of us has longer hair.
20. Point to something smaller than this (indicate a size).

Directions: Follow the instructions.

1. If you are wearing jewelry, smile.
2. If you have a pet, blink your eyes.
3. If you live alone, make a funny face.
4. If your hair is blond, stamp your foot.
5. If you sing in the shower, lift an arm.
6. If you like ice cream, scratch your ear.
7. If you have a brother, slap your knee.
8. If you are over 40, wink at me.
9. If you are an aunt or an uncle, swallow hard.
10. If you are a good speller, turn your head.
11. If you can play a musical instrument, make a humming noise.
12. If you like to cook, say *ah.*
13. If you have brown eyes, wiggle your fingers.
14. If you are tired, cough.
15. If you enjoy shopping, grab my hand.
16. If you speak two languages, close one eye.
17. If you wear glasses, point with one finger.
18. If you are left-handed, whistle.
19. If you have lived in the same place more than two years, laugh.
20. If it is before noon, lean forward.

Directions: Follow the instructions in order.

1. Scratch your head, then rub your stomach.
2. Tap your finger on the table, then on your knee.
3. Show me the palm of your left hand, then turn the hand over.
4. Blink your eyes, then close them.
5. Frown, then smile.
6. Put up three fingers, then your thumb.
7. Pretend you're snoring, then suddenly wake up.
8. Put your hand on your head, then rub it.
9. Make a sound like a fire engine, then whistle.
10. Look to your left, then to the ceiling.
11. Point to your elbow, then your chin.
12. Hold your nose, then clear your throat.
13. Put your arm in the air, then make a fist.
14. Count to three, then put up two fingers.
15. Moo like a cow, then meow like a cat.
16. Make a circle in the air, then an OK sign.
17. Open your eyes wide, then rub them.
18. Bend from the waist, then from the neck.
19. Wave good-bye, then yawn.
20. Hum a tune, then sing it.

Directions: Follow the instructions in order.

1. Nod your head yes, shake your head no, then raise your eyebrows.
2. Look to the ceiling, sigh, then look at the floor to your left.
3. Frown, put your tongue in your cheek, then smile showing your teeth.
4. Cross your arms, put your head on your chest, then put your left leg out in front of you.
5. Look over your right shoulder, tap your toe three times, then shake hands with me.
6. Make a fist, shake it toward the door, then put that same hand behind your back.
7. Stretch your arms toward the ceiling, put your hands on top of your head, then cover your ears with them.
8. Close your left eye, touch your right cheek with your left hand, then press that hand against your chin.
9. While seated, put one leg out straight, tap your leg two times, then cross that foot over the other leg.
10. Run your fingers through your hair, stick out your tongue, then touch your left ear.
11. Point to two things made of wood, pat your stomach, then point to two things made of plastic.
12. Cough, wipe under your nose with your hand, then pretend you have to sneeze.
13. Whistle, hum the beginning of "Happy Birthday," then say "ah."
14. Point to the younger one of us, put your hands on your hips, then squint your eyes.
15. Cross a hand to your opposite shoulder, bring your knees together, then take a deep breath.
16. Draw a circle in the air with a finger, touch your elbow with the same finger, then make an OK sign.
17. Put your arms out to the side, stretch them to the front, then put them over your head and quickly bring them down.
18. Spread your fingers apart, place them on top of your other hand, then remove the bottom hand and place it under your knee.
19. Tug on your ear with your left hand, blink your eyes twice, then place your pinky finger on your opposite elbow.
20. Place your hands on your knees, turn your hands over and back again, then scratch your neck.

If / Then Directions

Directions: Listen to the instructions, then follow them.

1. If a bull has three eyes, point to the floor. If it does not, scratch your nose.
2. If you are older than your father, put an arm behind your back. If you are not, put an arm in your lap.
3. If it is summer, wipe your brow. If it is not, touch the side of your nose.
4. If apples can be red or green, tap your toe twice. If they cannot, tap your hand twice.
5. If penguins live in warm climates, cover your mouth. If they do not, cover your eyes.
6. If slate is a rock, touch one thumb to the other thumb. If it is not, touch one thumb to its little finger.
7. If you need a prescription for vitamin pills, make a noise like a cow. If you do not, make a noise like a rooster.
8. If driveways and runways are the same thing, grab your earlobe. If they are not, grab your hair.
9. If dreams can wake you up, make a sound like you are snoring. If they cannot, make a sound like you are gagging.
10. If puddles can melt, turn your head to the left. If they cannot, turn your head to the right.
11. If there are 30 days in September, open your mouth as wide as you can. If there are not, curl back your lips and show your teeth.
12. If gingerbread is a type of bread, put your arm down at your side. If it is not, put your arm in the air.
13. If a mutual fund can be an investment, salute me. If it cannot, make an OK sign with your fingers.
14. If a country and a county are the same thing, put your hands on your hips. If they are not, put your hands on your head.
15. If trail mix is something to eat, sit up straight and put your shoulders back. If it is not, slouch down and round your shoulders forward.
16. If tobacco is good for you, lift your head back as far as it will go. If it is not, rest your chin on your chest.
17. If an area code has more than four numbers, cross your heart. If it does not, put your finger to your lips and say “shhh.”
18. If you were born in the twenty-first century, laugh out loud. If you were not, chuckle with your mouth closed.
19. If a turtleneck describes an animal, put one hand behind you. If it does not, wave to me.
20. If an expressway and a freeway are similar, point to your Adam’s apple. If they are not, point to your funny bone.

Directions: The sentence has two main elements. A yes/no question and an open-ended question follow each statement.

1. Breakfast is served. Is breakfast over? What is being served?
2. The grass was long. Is the hair long? What is long?
3. The rowboat sank. Did the sailboat sink? What sank?
4. The pizza is from Jet's. Is it from Domino's? What is from Jet's?
5. My wallet is missing. Are your keys missing? What is missing?
6. Heat the oven to 300 degrees. Are you using a microwave? What temperature do you want?
7. The kidnapper was caught. Is the criminal on the loose? Who was caught?
8. The eggs were overcooked. Were they too runny? What was overcooked?
9. The dog's name is Ralph. Is the pet named Rover? Who is Ralph?
10. The orchids are yellow. Are the flowers purple? What kind of flowers are they?
11. The poster was torn. Was it stained? What was torn?
12. The doctor has the flu. Does she have appendicitis? Who has the flu?
13. Raffle tickets are $10 each. Do they cost $5? What costs $10?
14. The brownies have nuts. Do they have nuts? What has nuts?
15. There was a fire in the warehouse. Was there a sale? What happened to the warehouse?
16. The jacket is downstairs. Is it outside? Where is the jacket?
17. The vase is cracked. Is it an urn? What is wrong with the vase?
18. The cat does not have fleas. Does it have fleas? What doesn't have fleas?
19. My ankle itches. Does your elbow itch? What's wrong with your ankle?
20. The senator is bald. Does he have hair? Who is bald?

Three-Element Statements

Directions: Each sentence has three elements. There is one question of each type (yes/no, multiple choice, and open-ended) for each sentence.

1. Nate flew to Buffalo.
   Did Nate go to Boise? Did Nate drive or fly? What was the man's name?
2. The drugstore opens at nine.
   Does the store close at nine? Is it a hardware or a drug store? What time does the store open?
3. My yellow T-shirt is ripped.
   Is the T-shirt yellow? Is the shirt dirty or ripped? What kind of clothing is it?
4. Invitations will be sent out Friday.
   Will letters be sent? Will they be sent out on Thursday or Friday? What will be sent?
5. Mike likes candy apples better than apple pie.
   Does Mike prefer pie? Is this about caramel apples or candy apples? Who likes the candy apples?
6. The spring broke on the garage door.
   Did the window break? Is the problem on the kitchen or the garage door? What broke?
7. The retriever caught the Frisbee.
   Did the dog drop it? Is it a rottweiler or a retriever? What did the dog catch?
8. Please mail the package at UPS.
   Should you mail it at the post office? Is it a letter or a package? Where do you take it?
9. The zipper broke on the suitcase.
   Was the zipper on a suitcase? Did the latch or the zipper break? What happened?
10. Soccer practice starts at 3:30.
    Does practice start at 3:00? Is it a game or a practice? What is the sport?
11. The muffins are tasteless and dry.
    Are the muffins good? Is the food cupcakes or muffins? What is wrong with the food?
12. Bob was arguing with the guard.
    Was Bob happy? Was Bob arguing with the guard or the owner? Who was mad?
13. The shredder needs four D batteries.
    Does it need four batteries? Does it need C or D batteries? What needs the batteries?
14. Tuesday the parking lot will close for repairs.
    Will the lot close to be repaved? Will the road or the parking lot close? When will it close?
15. Duffy's has great crab cakes and pies.
    Is it called Duffy's? Does it have good crab legs or crab cakes? What are the specialties?

16. Ed lost the home-insurance policy.
    Did Ted lose something? Did Ed lose a mortgage or an insurance policy? What did he lose?

17. The hinges on the cabinet are loose.
    Are the hinges loose? Are the hinges on the door or the cabinet? What is loose?

18. There is a loaf of garlic bread and two pieces of lasagna left.
    Will this serve two people? Is there leftover pizza or lasagna? What is for dinner?

19. The clearance sale ends tomorrow.
    Does the sale end today? Is it a clothing or a clearance sale? What happens tomorrow?

20. The Whitmans have two sons and a daughter.
    Do they have one son? Do they have more sons or daughters? What is the name of the family?

Add an Element

Directions: The words in brackets can be added to the statement to make it more complex. The open-ended question is based on the original sentence and could lead to more questions.

1. There is a [baby] blue jay on the [neighbor's] fence. What is on the fence?
2. The [cheddar] cheese is moldy [on the edges]. What is wrong with the cheese?
3. Ted jogged [two miles] in the [botanical] park. Where did Ted exercise?
4. The [gas] bill is due [a week from] Tuesday. When is it due?
5. The [soccer] team mascot is a [black] greyhound. What is the mascot?
6. [Computer] class starts at 7:30 [in room 30]. When does class start?
7. Your [reading] glasses are on the piano [bench]. Where are the glasses?
8. The [right] [rear] tire has a stone in it. What is wrong with the tire?
9. Alan has [a headache and] the [stomach] flu. Who has the flu?
10. The auditions [for *Survivor*] are at the arena [from 10:00 to 4:00]. What is happening at the arena?
11. Your parents are arriving [at 7:00] tomorrow [with their cat] to spend the weekend. Who is coming for a visit?
12. The [twin] Walker boys are very polite [and athletic]. What are the Walker boys like?
13. Please pick up [eight] [jelly] donuts on your way home [from Kelly's]. What should you pick up?
14. She canceled the [surprise] party [for her sister]. What did she cancel?
15. The [35 percent] discount coupon [for Eddie Bauer] expires on Friday. What expires?
16. The [chicken] [rice] soup was not hot. How was the soup?
17. [Yesterday] I visited George after his [hernia] operation. Who did you visit?
18. Carolyn postponed the [staff] meeting [until Thursday]. What did Carolyn postpone?
19. [Next] Wednesday all [gold] jewelry is on sale [at Tapper's]. What is on sale?
20. I lost ten pounds [in three weeks] on the chicken [and chocolate] diet. How much did you lose?

Directions: Listen to the information and answer the question.

1. An elephant's trunk can hold two gallons of water.
   How much water can the trunk hold?

2. Mohammed is the most popular male name in the world.
   What is the most popular man's name?

3. In 1896, the world's first escalator was introduced in Coney Island, New York.
   What was introduced?

4. Seventy-five percent of the people in the United States live on 2 percent of the land.
   What percentage of Americans live on 2 percent of the land?

5. Camel-hair brushes are really made from squirrel hair.
   What type of brush is made from squirrel hair?

6. Cows give more milk when they listen to music.
   Why would music be playing in a barn?

7. Toy dog breeds live an average of seven years longer than large breeds.
   What type of breed lives longest?

8. Tae Kwon Do began in Korea around 50 B.C.
   What started in B.C.?

9. Hummingbirds flap their wings 50–75 beats per second.
   How fast do the wings beat?

10. As of 2005, the world's longest roller coaster is 1.54 miles and located in Japan.
    How long is the longest roller coaster?

11. An adult tooth releases a chemical that dissolves the root of a baby tooth so that it loosens and eventually falls out.
    Why does a baby tooth fall out?

12. Every time you sneeze, your heart stops and you cannot sneeze with your eyes open.
    What happens when you sneeze?

13. Sap travels in and out of a tree, not up and down the bark.
    How does sap move in a tree?

14. It is the bacteria on your skin that causes the odor from perspiration.
    What causes perspiration odor?

15. Before the golf tee was patented in 1899, people hit golf balls off a small pile of wet sand.
    What did golfers use before tees?

16. At one time, yams in Mexico were used in the production of steroids and birth control pills.
    What were yams used for?

17. Ancient Egyptians thought it was good luck to step into your home with your left foot first.
    What did Egyptians think was good luck?

18. The richest country in the world is Switzerland and the poorest is Mozambique.
    What are the richest and poorest countries?

19. One remedy for dark circles under the eyes is to rub almond oil in the area before going to bed.
    How can you help get rid of dark circles under your eyes?

20. Instead of a covering of scales, sharks have denticles that are sharp enough to tear your skin.
    What are denticles like?

Directions: Listen to the sentence, and then answer the question with yes or no.

1. Bob was tied up all day. Was he busy?
2. Lynn is really run-down. Is Lynn hurt?
3. The concert started on the dot. Did it start on time?
4. The prisoner is at large. Is he behind bars?
5. Joe flew off the handle. Was he upset?
6. Take it with a grain of salt. Should you believe it?
7. He's nuts about ice cream. Does he like it?
8. She eats like a bird. Does she eat worms?
9. The practical joke backfired. Did it go over well?
10. Barb hit the sack at 9:00. Did she go to bed?
11. The drinks were on the house. Were they paid for?
12. They will tie the knot on Saturday. Are they going sailing?
13. The comedian brought down the house. Was he funny?
14. Once in a blue moon I have a hot fudge sundae. Do I have it often?
15. Lee swallowed his pride and apologized. Was he eating?
16. They worked around the clock until the job was done. Did they work all night?
17. I had to pull some strings to get tickets. Was it easy to get tickets?
18. She looks like a million dollars. Is she looking green?
19. The groom arrived just in the nick of time. Did he come too late?
20. Jogging is not my cup of tea. Do I like jogging?

True or False

Directions: Indicate if the sentence is true or false.

1. Yardsticks grow on trees.
2. Croutons are made from bread.
3. A Sudoku is a small Japanese car.
4. A rhinestone is a natural gem.
5. Publicity can be good or bad.
6. Cider is made from oranges.
7. Your skull protects your brain.
8. A rubber band can stretch to fit around any shape.
9. An example of a prank could be to put sugar in a salt shaker.
10. Children must be baptized before they can enter the public schools.
11. Mortgage rates can be fixed or adjustable.
12. Botox injections are given to provide protection from botulism poisoning.
13. Pinocchio is known for having a nose that grows.
14. An iPod is a vegetable.
15. In a table setting, the knife and spoon are placed together.
16. Food that is labeled kosher has been blessed by a rabbi or a priest.
17. A thermometer controls the temperature in a room.
18. In-laws are relatives you get through marriage.
19. Arthritis is caused by general muscle weakness.
20. You could have fondue for an appetizer, main course, or dessert.

Directions: Listen to the two sentences, then indicate if they mean about the same or not.

1. The cake is very rich. The very rich eat cake.
2. That's hard to believe. I can't believe it.
3. He made money in the stock market. He inherited money and stocks.
4. John is always on time for meetings. John is never late to meetings.
5. The jewelry box was kept in a safe. The jewelry box was safe.
6. He just moved here from Cleveland. He used to live in Cleveland.
7. I enjoyed the party but didn't like the food. I enjoyed the food but didn't like the party.
8. I didn't get much sleep last night. I have to get some sleep tonight.
9. John never missed a game. John went to all the games.
10. The boxer stopped at every tree. There was a box under every tree.
11. All baby chicks are cute. All cute chicks are babies.
12. Throw the anchor overboard. Throw the board over the anchor.
13. Everyone except Jenny likes cherries. Jenny likes cherries.
14. Even though the trailer was heated, I was cold. I was not feeling the heat in the trailer.
15. Ron is a good doctor. Ron needs a good doctor.
16. People can feel older than they look. People can look older than they feel.
17. I like wheat bread much better than rye. I don't care for rye bread.
18. The dog growled at the stranger. The strange dog growled.
19. Three blue boxes of soap are in the cabinet. Three boxes of soap are in the blue cabinet.
20. The sun was out only one day this week. Most of the week it was cloudy.

Change a Word

Receptive: Sentence Comprehension

Directions: There is one word in each sentence that makes it incorrect. Listen to the sentence, then indicate what word to change so the sentence makes sense.

1. I replaced the burned-out bulb with a broken one.
2. She got hives from the ATM machine.
3. Bruises from the fire covered 80 percent of his body.
4. After rubbing in the coat of shellac, the car's finish glistened in the sun.
5. The bears flew south for the winter.
6. The boat sailed out of the intersection.
7. The robin dug for acorns in the ground.
8. My new Teflon-lined gloves should keep my hands nice and warm.
9. The noise from your smoking kept me awake.
10. Mike will turn 50 years old on September 34.
11. After two weeks of no attention, the lawn really needed vacuuming.
12. The specialty of the sushi restaurant is eggplant parmesan.
13. Health professionals say it is important to drink eight quarts of water daily.
14. She put the Jell-O in the closet to set.
15. University of Michigan has its spring break the third week in July.
16. The farmer put the crows out to pasture.
17. The police officer presented me with an award for speeding.
18. Most people need between seven and eight minutes of sleep per night.
19. The new hybrid cars use a combination of electricity and coffee as fuel.
20. I was so hungry I couldn't eat another bite.

Directions: Listen to the sentence, then answer the question.

1. The blue scarf is cheaper than the red one. Which scarf costs less?
2. The handles on the brass pot are made of wood. What part is wooden?
3. Two large branches blew off the elm during the storm. What kind of tree was it?
4. The air was hot in the bedroom but cool in the kitchen. Which room was cool?
5. The Utah state trooper pulled over the truck with the Iowa plates. Where was the trooper from?
6. The red-checkered napkins looked nice on the white tablecloth. What color were the napkins?
7. On the way to our cabin, we stopped at a fruit and vegetable stand. Where were we going?
8. Hallman's clothing store received a shipment of shoes last week. What kind of store is it?
9. The news report said that six persons drowned and three were rescued. How many died?
10. The gifted Spanish pianist was only 13 years old. What was the player's nationality?
11. I'm wearing my black sweater with tan pants. What color is the sweater?
12. The city council passed a parking ordinance by a vote of 10 to 4. Who voted on the issue?
13. The emerald ring was claimed by Mrs. King after 10 days. What kind of ring was it?
14. Tim McGraw had three curtain calls after his concert. How many curtain calls were there?
15. Cameo pins were hot sellers at the coin, jewelry, and antiques show. What was the popular item?
16. Of the four furniture polishes, Tipton's Tonic worked the best. How many were tested?
17. The tomatoes aren't ripe yet, but the lima beans are. Which are ready to eat?
18. My handyman fell in my driveway and broke his wrist. Who hurt himself?
19. An auto company recalled 5,000 trucks for an oil gauge problem. How many were recalled?
20. They have a great view of the lake from the bay window in the dining room. What can they see?

Directions: Listen to the sentence, then answer the question with yes or no.

1. The reservations were for six at 8:00. Were eight people expected?
2. I have had chicken pox but not mumps. Have I had mumps?
3. The card shop is open from 1:00 to 4:00 on Sunday. Is it open in the afternoon?
4. Plastic sheeting is laid down before the gravel. Does the gravel go on first?
5. The cable goes from the TV to the VCR. Are the VCR and the TV connected?
6. There is a detour for the Park Street Bridge. Can you drive on the bridge?
7. The game went two extra innings and delayed the start of the nightly news. Did the game go into overtime?
8. Kate is going to tour Jake's art studio. Is Jake the artist?
9. The new computer will come by FedEx. Will it be delivered?
10. The Lions Club meets the second Tuesday of every month. Does it meet twice a month?
11. My white shirt is in the wash, so I'll wear my navy one. Do I have a white shirt?
12. Laura invited Carol to the Heart Association meeting. Is Laura the guest?
13. My doctor sees patients Tuesday through Friday. Does my doctor see patients on Thursday?
14. The left rear tire of a car in the parking lot was flat. Was the front tire flat?
15. Don't take the medication on a full stomach. Should the pill be taken before eating a big meal?
16. After the planning meeting we'll go to an Italian restaurant. Will we eat first?
17. They are behind three months in rent. Do they owe money?
18. I bought 40 envelopes, a dozen greeting cards, and some gift wrap. Did I buy a dozen envelopes?
19. The raccoon sat on a log and ate an orange. Was he sitting in the water?
20. The pumpkin weighed over 25 pounds. Did it weigh more than 10 pounds?

Directions: Listen to the sentence, then answer the question.

1. Bob and John followed Mary into the store. Who went first?
2. We drove from Spruceville up the coast to Linwood. Which place is farther north?
3. The blue jay landed between the robin and the sparrow. Which bird was in the middle?
4. The drugstore is closed between midnight and 7:00. What hours is it open?
5. Although the portions were huge, the food was nutritious. Was the food good for you?
6. Jake ate his egg before the sausage but after the toast. What did he eat first?
7. It is 5:00 and there are three hours before the play starts but one and a half hours before we have to leave home. What time do we leave?
8. The bill is due the first of the month and finance charges accrue from the fifth until payment is received. How can you avoid finance charges?
9. The new CEO has been with the company for 15 years—eight in engineering and seven in marketing. Where did he spend more time?
10. Although he was sentenced to six years in prison, he was released on parole four years early. How many years was he in prison?
11. In a tragic fire, the father and two children died, while the mother and three older children escaped without injury. How many were in the family?
12. Sara Hill's office manager gave the message that her lawyer had called. Is Ms. Hill the attorney?
13. I need to stop at the drugstore before the hardware store but not the grocery store even though it's on the way. How many stops will I make?
14. If I knew that Barb didn't have insurance, I wouldn't have lent her my car. Did I let her borrow my car?
15. The bus tour began in Philadelphia with stops in Manhattan and Atlantic City. How many states did the bus go through?
16. The daffodils bloomed a week earlier than the tulips and two weeks later than the crocuses. What bloomed last?
17. The photograph shows Nancy Reagan standing to the left of Laura Bush, who is to the left of Barbara Bush. Who is in the middle?
18. The puppy needs to be vaccinated before we can get a license, but it needs a shot for worms before it can be vaccinated. In what order do things need to happen?
19. Mr. Boyd has to take a pink pill before each meal, a white pill twice a day, and two capsules morning and night. How many pills does he take a day?
20. While Alan is gone, Bill will take care of Fred, his dog, and Bart, his cat. Who owns the pets?

Mixed Questions 2

Directions: Listen to the sentence, then answer the question.

1. The store manager claims he will beat any competitor's price or he'll give you $500 or a new grill.
   What will the manager do to avoid paying a customer $500?
2. The wedding will take place six weeks after Labor Day.
   What season will the wedding be in?
3. A physician can prescribe medicine but not necessarily operate, but a surgeon can do both.
   Who can write a prescription as well as perform an appendectomy?
4. The Golf League requires that if you can't golf, you must give 24-hours' notice and arrange for a substitute or you forfeit the game.
   What could you do if you got sick the afternoon of your golf night?
5. The article's advice is to eliminate sweets, cut down on red meat, and increase your intake of fruits and vegetables.
   What was the goal of the advice?
6. I bought a belt the day before yesterday and I tried to return it today, but the store is closed because it is Sunday.
   What day did I buy the belt?
7. Although he was not incarcerated, he had to pay court costs and do 100 hours of community service.
   Was he found guilty?
8. The editor wanted to keep the murder quiet, so he buried the story in the sports section.
   Did the editor kill someone?
9. The artist will paint from 10:00 to 12:00, then again from 4:00 to 8:00.
   How much time will he take off?
10. It takes twice as long to drive to the theater as to walk and half as long to take a shuttle.
    What is the fastest way to get there?
11. Many years ago, we went to London on the *Queen Mary.*
    Did we meet royalty?
12. Cher, Madonna, Nemo, and Elton John will be participating in the concert.
    Who is the odd one in this group?
13. After searching 40 minutes for a missing ring, Joan commented, "That sure was fun."
    What emotion was she experiencing?
14. There will be some bruising around the stitches but there will be minimal scarring.
    What might have happened?

15. The sign says “Children must be at least 4'10" before they can ride.”
    Where would the sign be?

16. He kept pushing a button and saw a commercial, then a weather report, then a newscast.
    What kind of button was it?

17. The park dedication ceremony will be Saturday from 12:00 to 4:00. If it rains, it will be rescheduled to next Sunday from 1:00 to 2:00.
    How many days will the ceremony be postponed if it rains?

18. The leftover steak was wrapped in foil.
    Can you put the whole thing in the microwave?

19. If it weren’t for hairstyles and clothing, you would not be able to tell the boys apart.
    What else could you guess about the boys?

20. The coupon was for a 30 percent discount on two 40-ounce bottles.
    How many bottles do you need to buy?

Directions: Listen to the sentence, then answer the questions.

1. If you could take a pound of cobwebs and spread them out in a straight line, they would wind around the earth two times.
   How long would the webs extend? How many cobwebs would you need?

2. Every time he sings a concert, Luciano Pavarotti carries a bent nail in his top pocket for good luck.
   Is Pavarotti superstitious? What does he carry?

3. Kool-Aid was developed in 1927 by a chemist from Nebraska and it is still popular, with about 17 gallons consumed every second of every day.
   How much Kool-Aid is consumed? Who developed it?

4. A bristlecone pine on Mt. Wheeler in Nevada is thought to be the world's oldest tree.
   What kind of tree is it? What state is it in?

5. Spittlebugs are insects that are about one-half inch long and look like very tiny frogs.
   What size are the bugs? What is the name of the bugs?

6. In 1976, red M&M's were removed from the market because of a scare about red dye No. 2, but they were brought back in 1987 because the company received so much mail asking for their return.
   What color was not produced for a few years? Why not?

7. Florida is not just an eastern state, because portions of it are farther west then the eastern edge of Wisconsin.
   What is unusual about Florida? What other state was mentioned?

8. It is true that you can tell the temperature in Fahrenheit by counting the number of a cricket's chirps in 14 seconds and then adding 32 to that number.
   What information can crickets give you? What do you listen to and for how long?

9. A Slinky is made with 80 feet of wire, and in 1999, on its 50th anniversary, the Slinky was commemorated on a postage stamp.
   If a Slinky were unwound, how long would it be? Is the Slinky older than you are?

10. In 1996, Pepsi had to cancel its giveaway campaign when it realized it had underestimated by $60 million how many people would enter and win.
    What was the company's error? What was the name of the company?

11. Before Beethoven sat down to write music, he would pour a pitcher of ice water over his head because he felt it would stimulate his brain.
    How did Beethoven prepare himself to be creative? Why did he do it?

12. The Frisbee was named after the Frisbee Baking Company in Connecticut because their metal baking tins had been used for years by Yale students who tossed them to each other.
    How did the Frisbee get its name? What was the original item that was used?

13. In 1987, an airline saved $40,000 by eliminating one olive from each salad served in first class.
    Would passengers likely be upset by this cost-saving measure? How much was saved?

14. Opossums will eat anything, they don't fight, they have a top speed of 1.7 mph, and they have almost the smallest brain-to-body ratio of all land mammals.
    What do opossums eat? How fast do they move?

15. Poison ivy is more toxic in the spring and summer, and clothing can remain contaminated for many years.
    When is poison ivy worse? What should you do with contaminated clothing?

16. A 730-pound mako shark was once caught near the Bahamas with a whole 120-pound swordfish, including the sword, in its stomach.
    How many pounds was the shark? What had it swallowed?

17. Flamingoes get their pink color from eating blue-green algae called Spirulina that produces a red pigment in flamingo feathers.
    What do pink flamingoes eat? Why do some flamingoes look very pink?

18. In the early years of the space program, the United States spent a million dollars developing a pen that could write upside-down and in zero gravity, while the Russian space program had their astronauts use pencils.
    What did the U.S. develop? Who do you think had the better idea?

19. In the 1970s, Gary Dahl became a millionaire after about one-and-a-quarter million Americans spent $3.95 each to buy his pet rock.
    When was the pet rock most popular? How much did it cost?

20. The hottest pepper, a red Savina habanero, can be detected by your taste buds even when just a very tiny bit is added to a 700-pound vat of sauce.
    What is the name of the hottest pepper? Would you like a drop of it on your tongue?

Directions: Listen to the sentence, then answer the questions.

1. Katy watched *The Apprentice* until 10:00, read *Newsweek* until 10:45, let the dog out and in, had a glass of water, and turned off the light at 11:05.
   What did Katy read? When was "lights out"? What did she do after bringing in the dog?

2. The recipe called for adding the oil and vanilla after sifting the flour and baking soda together, then folding in the nuts at the end.
   What do you put in first? What do you fold in? What do you sift together?

3. As CEO of Tech Business Corporation, I am pleased to announce that on March 28, George Clarkson from Solutions for Business will be joining us as our chief financial officer.
   When will the change happen? What company will he be joining? Who is announcing this?

4. The salad dressings are in aisle six on the right on the bottom two shelves below the pickles.
   What aisle is mentioned? What other product is nearby? What are you looking for?

5. The first buffet table has omelets to order, then the table on the right is a salad bar, while the table on the left has a cheese tray at the end but starts with all kinds of fruits and rolls.
   What is on the table on the left? What is on the first table? Where is the salad bar?

6. Your opera tickets are for the third and fourth seats from the end of row F on the second mezzanine.
   What are the tickets for? What two seats do you have? What row are they in?

7. Recent renovations on this 1965 colonial include a new efficiency furnace, central air, the addition of a first-floor bath and laundry room, and a bay window in the living room.
   What type of home is it? What is new in the living room? What two rooms were added?

8. Red Lobster is located in the Sears wing on the third floor before you get to Sharper Image and after you pass Mrs. Fields.
   What place are you looking for? What two places is it between? What floor is it on?

9. Pull down the Format menu, click *line*; click *spacing*, and under *line spacing* click on the words *at least* and *12 points*.
   What menu do you pull down? Where is the *at least* and *12 points* located?

10. Before you fill out paperwork in Human Resources, you need to give your application to the supervisor who is down the hall in the third office on your left.
    What do you do first? Where is the supervisor's office? What department are you in?

11. Darryl, don't leave until you say good-bye to Taylor and his cousin Kelly who are visiting with Kimberly, whose husband you played golf with last week.
    Who are visiting? Who did Darryl play golf with? Who is the cousin?

12. Please bring me my glasses which are probably on the nightstand, but you should check the kitchen counter or my purse before you go upstairs.
    Where should you check first? What are you looking for? Where is the purse?

13. What a day—I had two people show up for a 10:00 appointment and this was after my 9:00 didn't come and then I was the only one who showed up for an 11:00 meeting.
    What appointment did not show up? When was the meeting? What happened at 10:00?

14. For sale: 2004 pearl-gray Mercury Mountaineer with moonroof, 25,500 miles, excellent condition, and fold-down third seat.
    What color is it? How many miles are on it? What year and type of car is it?

15. Barky, the cocker, likes to play with his food so he should be fed last, while Molly, the retriever, gulps down her food so she can get back to her squeaky toys.
    Who eats slowly? Who likes squeaky toys? What are the dogs' names?

16. It's hard to imagine that just three years ago Tom was only up to my shoulder and today Tim, his younger brother by two years, is taller than both of us.
    Who is the tallest? When was Tom up to your shoulder? Who is the oldest?

17. The 14th annual antique Trade Cards Convention will be held at the Eagle Hotel in Bloomfield, Michigan, the weekend of November 21–23.
    What type of convention is it? Where are the rooms? What are the dates?

18. Kevin was married to Lillian, but he was really in love with Brooke, who had his child, but she was trying to get Elliott to marry her so she told him the child was his.
    Who had Kevin's child? Who does Brooke love? Who is the married couple?

19. The leader board shows three golfers tied for the lead at five under par with four holes left to play, while Tiger is already in the clubhouse with four under par waiting to see what happens.
    How many holes do the leaders have to play? What is Tiger's score? How many are in the lead and what are their scores?

20. The Lockwood-Lincoln Foundation provides scholarships to deserving individuals who will be attending Lawrence University and majoring in neurology and who have volunteered in a senior center, live on an island, and have an uncle in the furniture business.
    Who is giving the scholarships? What will be the major of the recipient? Name another criteria individuals have to meet.

Directions: Listen to the sentence, then answer the questions.

1. Please pick up the laundry by 5:00 and the dog from the groomer by 6:00, buy a book of stamps, figure out what you want for dinner and pick it up on your way home.
   Where do you have to be by 6:00? What's for dinner?

2. Lunch at Peabody's has been changed from Thursday to Wednesday and from 11:30 to 12:15, so be sure to call Mary at extension 20 if you still want to reserve a seat.
   When is lunch at Peabody's? Why do you need to call Mary?

3. Office hours are from 8:00 to 4:30 on Monday and Wednesday and from 10:00 to 7:30 on Tuesday and Friday.
   What are the hours on Wednesday? What day is the office closed?

4. Mix three cups of water with one cup of liquid soap, one cup of ginger ale, one quarter cup of honey, and two tablespoons of oatmeal.
   How much ginger ale do you use? Which ingredient would you not want to eat?

5. We need you to fill out the bottom half of form 7346 with your name and address, social security number, date of birth, and policy number, and on the second page write a detailed written account of the missing items.
   What is the form number? What do you put on page two?

6. Amy has to get to Scouts at 5:00, so she needs to be picked up from soccer after Natalie, who will have finished cheerleading practice and needs to get to her job at Wendy's.
   What happens at 5:00? Who works at Wendy's?

7. I would like to order a chocolate sheet cake with white icing to feed 40 for next Wednesday decorated with pastel-colored flowers and the message, "Good luck Barbara, we will miss you" written on it.
   What kind of cake are you ordering? Why are you ordering a cake?

8. Let's meet in Kroger's parking lot at 8:30 and I will pack a lunch for everyone if you will bring beverages and some dessert—and don't forget to bring four 20 percent off admission coupons.
   What will the speaker bring? When and where do you meet?

9. Tell the guard you are the parents of Cadet Kelly in Military Hall on south campus and are visiting but that first you need directions to get to the commissary so you can bring the supplies she wants.
   Where does the cadet live? What directions do you need?

10. I would like two medium pizzas—one with pepperoni, mushrooms, and extra cheese and the other vegetarian but no mushrooms and a large Greek salad with no dressing.
    Name the ingredients on one of the pizzas. Besides pizza, what is the order?

11. Northwest Airlines flight 648 is due to depart at 8:32 P.M. but will be delayed by at least 45 minutes because of a delayed departure out of Philadelphia due to bad weather.
    What is the flight number of the delayed plane? Why is it delayed?

12. Please put any items for the Scouts in the bag provided on your porch by 9:30 next Saturday and staple a completed form to the top of the bag if you want a tax receipt sent to you.
    Who is collecting the bags? Why would you staple something to the bag?

13. To participate in the exchange, bring a wrapped gift with a value of no more than $10 that would appeal to a child between ages five and eight and put a girl's gift in the red barrel and a boy's gift in the yellow barrel.
    How much should you spend? What goes in the red barrel?

14. Take Maple Road to Telegraph, turn right and go north for three miles until you come to Hickory Grove Road, where you turn left and then right into the third driveway.
    How far do you go on Telegraph? What street do you turn left on?

15. Our fee for mowing the yard is $24 per week, which includes edging every other week, blowing the walkways, and eight applications of spray fertilizer for $27 each for a special price of $280 for the season.
    How many applications of fertilizer do you get? How much is the weekly mowing and what does it include?

16. Tom should have lots of liquids and soft foods but not any products that contain beef or soy for the next two weeks, and he should take a B-vitamin and an iron supplement and not lift anything heavier than a half-gallon of milk.
    What should Tom avoid for two weeks? What supplement should he take?

17. We are leaving at 5:00 A.M. and will cross the border into Canada at Port Huron and cross back into the states at Niagara Falls, where we'll take the New York Thruway to the Mass Pike and get off at Sturbridge in time for dinner.
    Where will we cross into Canada? Where will we have dinner? What time are we leaving?

18. The 14-inch chain is 18-carat gold with a platinum claw clasp, and the pendant has a center 1.2-carat tanzanite surrounded by 12 faceted diamonds.
    How long is the chain? What stones are in the pendant?

19. The three messages are to call Lindsay about working for her tomorrow night, Borders has your special-order book, *Aphasia for Dummies*, at the main desk, and your accountant wants to know when you purchased Ford stock and at what price.
    What was the second message? What stock was mentioned and why?

20. The X-ray department needs to change your Saturday morning appointment at 8:30 to Wednesday the 23rd at 4:30; please return this call to confirm the change with us.
    When was the original appointment? What kind of appointment is it?

Directions: Listen to the information and answer the questions.

1. The VISA bill showed purchases at Rite-Aid, Home Depot, Nordstrom, Festivities, and TJ Maxx.
   Which place is not a national chain? What was the first store?

2. As we travel to Chapel Hill, we will pass through Mansfield, Huntington, Jefferson, Cherokee, and Asheville.
   Where are we going? What are the last two places we will go through?

3. The Fit and Fun Gym has a number of crunch machines, balance balls, leg press machines, elliptical trainers, and resistance bands.
   What machines are provided? What is the name of the gym?

4. Stack the towels in the following order: sage green, sky blue, cream, white with rose trim, and yellow.
   What colors are on the trimmed towel? What color is on the bottom of the stack?

5. The movies that have been nominated for the Animated Family-Friendly Award are: *Madascar*, *Shrek*, *A Bug's Life*, *Finding Nemo*, and *Fantasia*.
   What are the one-word titles? What is the name of the award?

6. The main ingredients for the chicken casserole are a box of wild rice, a bunch of asparagus, a can of cream of celery soup, one chopped-up onion, and a pint of sliced mushrooms.
   What kind of casserole is it? What kind of soup is used?

7. The people at Katy's going-away party were Tom and Ann, Jason and Jill, Nicole, the Engles, and her parents.
   Why was there a party? Who was not part of a twosome?

8. The pets we had growing up were Scruffy the mutt, Potsy the parrot, Hopper the bunny, Squeaker the guinea pig, and Harry the turtle.
   What were the two pet names beginning with S? What are the five kinds of pets?

9. The ingredients in the yogurt are in order: cultured pasteurized nonfat milk, naturally milled sugar, natural vanilla flavor, live active cultures, and pectin.
   What is the main ingredient? What flavor is the yogurt?

10. The islands the ship will be stopping at are Belize, Grenada, Jamaica, Martinique, and Aruba.
    What islands begin with the first two letters of the alphabet? What is the third island?

11. In order to bring the house up to code, the following problems need to be fixed: leaking roof, broken bathroom tiles, ceiling cracks, dripping bath faucets, and rotting deck wood.
    What is the second problem? What problems are outside?

12. The specials of the day are turkey Reuben sandwich, salmon Caesar salad, pasta Alfredo, spring vegetable soup, and turtle cheesecake.
    What is the salad special? What dishes would be served hot?

13. The guests this week on Letterman include actress Julia Roberts, Senator John McCain, author Scott Turow, producer George Clooney, and comedian Chris Rock.
    What senator is appearing? Who is the fourth guest?

14. The coffee flavors of the day are mocha latte, cinnamon hazelnut, chocolate raspberry, decaf organic Ethiopian blend, and eye-opener breakfast blend.
    Which one is decaffeinated? What blend will have a nutty flavor?

15. The new officers of the Press Club are treasurer Susan Blake, secretary Tony Case, member-at-large Ellen Howell, vice-president Ginger John, and president Lydia Kirkwood.
    What are the first names of the officers? Who is member-at-large?

16. The house at 93 Country Road is a 4 bedroom, 3.5 bath ranch with an updated kitchen with granite countertops, a large great room with 2-story fireplace, and a completely finished walk-out lower level with its own kitchen and bath.
    Describe the kitchen. How many baths does the home have?

17. My great-great-grandfather was Ezekiel, my great grandfather was Jeremiah, my grandfather was Winston, my father is Robert, and I am Rob Junior.
    What is the name of the oldest ancestor? What is the grandfather's name?

18. Before the in-laws arrive, we have to put away the paper piles, clean out an area of the closet, clean the toilet and shower, clear off the nightstand, put out a water pitcher and glasses, and get a nightlight for the room.
    What needs to be done in the bedroom? Why do you need to clean?

19. The next two weekends are very full with Saturday morning volunteering at the recycling center, Annie's birthday party at 6:30, Sunday brunch at Applebee's followed by a 2:00 tee time, and the following weekend I have a tax seminar in Ann Arbor all day Saturday.
    When are there open hours during the first weekend? What kind of seminar is scheduled?

20. We only have five more things to get for the scavenger hunt, and they are a map of a state beginning with N, a penny from the 1970s, a red baseball cap, a key ring in the shape of a fruit, and a shopping bag from a place that starts with the letter *C*.
    What type of coin do you need? What needs to begin with the letter N?

Inferential Information 1

Receptive: Sentence Comprehension

Directions: Listen to the sentence, then answer the question with yes or no.

1. Nancy grabbed her purse and raced out the door. Do you think she was in a hurry?
2. It was a perfect summer day. Was it cloudy?
3. The paper is delivered between 5 and 7 A.M. Is it there before most people go to work?
4. Puddles were everywhere, and mud covered the sidewalks. Was it a dry spell?
5. The wet clothes were taken out of the washing machine. Were they clean?
6. Mr. Black called AAA to have his car towed. Can he drive his car?
7. My luggage was not transferred to the correct flight. Was I traveling by train?
8. Don had the sleeves lengthened and the pants shortened. Is this about clothing?
9. Mom's blue Ford is parked next to the red Pontiac. Do I own a blue car?
10. The woman had a walking cast and was using crutches. Did she hurt her shoulder?
11. The stray cat takes food from my garbage can. Does the cat belong to me?
12. Joan cried when Ed gave her a diamond necklace. Was she happy?
13. He blew out the candles while the others sang a song. Was it a special occasion?
14. Bob ordered two cheese pizzas to go. Is he planning to sit there and eat?
15. The Dodgers put an end to the Cubs' winning streak last night. Did the Dodgers win the game?
16. She handed the man his reward money as he returned her ring. Was she buying the ring?
17. As she walked, she buttoned up her coat and put on her gloves. Was she cold?
18. The doctor said I could eat whatever I felt like. Does the doctor want me on a strict diet?
19. The waves and salt water against her legs felt good. Was she at a zoo?
20. The doors and windows of the store were boarded up. Was it open for business?

Inferential Information 2

Directions: Listen to the sentence, then indicate the correct answer from the choices.

1. I'm going to wash clothes. Do I need detergent or shampoo?
2. The pizza was burned around the edges. Was it undercooked or overcooked?
3. The rock struck the glass and it shattered. Did the rock or the glass break?
4. I haven't a clue about who took the dollar Ann laid on the table. Did Ann take the dollar or not?
5. She cleaned the floor with soap and water. Did she wash or sweep it?
6. I haven't seen hide nor hair of Erik. Is he around or not?
7. He slammed his foot on the brake. Did he stop slowly or suddenly?
8. The basket overflowed with fresh vegetables. Was the basket full or nearly empty?
9. The road was filled with potholes. Should you drive fast or slow?
10. Everyone but my niece Jane went to the party. Did Jane attend or not?
11. The paint will not be fully dry for 36 hours. Will the paint take more or less than a day to dry?
12. Pears, peaches, and raisins were in the salad. Was it a fruit or vegetable salad?
13. He hit the jackpot in Reno. Did he get money or get into a fight?
14. The Smiths say the one thing they don't need right now is another pet. Would you surprise them with a kitten or a casserole?
15. The path through the woods was narrow, winding, and poorly marked. Would it be easy or hard to follow?
16. The power went out, so we lit a bunch of candles. Was this during the day or evening?
17. The audience wanted to hear the group's old hits. Was this a music or sporting event?
18. The foundation is laid, and the frame will be constructed soon. Is a car or a house being built?
19. The news story was obviously slanted toward the victims of violent crimes. Did the story focus on those who committed the crimes or those against whom the crimes were committed?
20. I'm sick and tired of hearing about how the government spends our tax money. Am I upset or ill?

Drawing Conclusions 1

Receptive: Sentence Comprehension

Directions: Listen to the sentence, then indicate the correct answer from the choices.

1. The bellhop took our bags to the room. Were we at a school or a hotel?
2. Jan designs jewelry for relaxation. Does she do this for fun or for a profit?
3. The children hung their wet suits on the line to dry. Had they been swimming or reading?
4. Nancy's cake has 24 candles on it. Is it a birthday or a wedding?
5. Glen is standing next to Sam. Is Sam behind or beside Glen?
6. They warmed their hands in front of the roaring fire. Were they probably cold or hot?
7. Dan took off his sweatsuit and put on his pajamas. Was he getting ready to exercise or go to bed?
8. The cat was rubbing against my legs and purring. Was it happy or upset?
9. John's mouth ached, and it hurt him to chew on the left side. Should he call a dentist or a doctor?
10. The host put out bowls of pretzels, nuts, and chips. Was he serving dessert or snacks?
11. Art is searching the web for information. Is he online or on foot?
12. The box was wrapped in colorful paper and had a big white bow. Was it a package or a plant?
13. She made an appointment for a manicure and a trim. Did she call a beauty salon or a lawn service?
14. She recorded the patient's vital signs. Was she in a store or a hospital?
15. These shoes squeeze my toes. Do I need to buy a smaller or a larger size?
16. He dribbled the ball down the court before shooting. Was he playing basketball or baseball?
17. Carol gave the number of the restaurant to her babysitter. Was she coming in or going out?
18. As the starter gun fired, the runners took off. Was it a car race or a foot race?
19. She opened the door, and he held out a heart-shaped box of candy and a red rose. Was it Labor Day or Valentine's Day?
20. The shopping center has escalators and stairs. Does it have more than one floor?

Drawing Conclusions 2

Directions: Listen to the sentence, then indicate the correct answer from the choices.

1. Some of the plant's leaves have turned yellowish and brittle. Does it need fertilizer or water?
2. Laura is two weeks overdue. Does she have an overdue book or baby?
3. Please hold and I'll transfer you to the main office. Would this be said in person or over the phone?
4. I'd like two scoops with sprinkles. Is this about sand or ice cream?
5. Take an alternate route on I-75 south until further notice. Is this about a detour or a store closing?
6. Pile three cups of thinly sliced apples into an unbaked crust. Are you making pie or pizza?
7. I'll get my racket and meet you on the court in 15 minutes. Are they playing golf or tennis?
8. Ties are on the second floor by the escalator. Is this in a store or an office?
9. I'll have an egg roll and almond chicken. Is this at a Mexican or Chinese restaurant?
10. This old T-shirt is too tight. Have you lost or gained weight?
11. All he ever reads is the stocks and sports. Does he read novels or papers?
12. This baby has 300 horsepower and a V-8 engine. Is he talking about a person or a car?
13. I began to understand the plot in the third chapter. Is this about a book or a movie?
14. Do you want ketchup or mustard? Are you eating a salad or a burger?
15. Where do you keep your Q-tips? Would this be in a bathroom or a kitchen?
16. Beads of sweat were dripping down his back. Was he hot or cold?
17. I have a new e-mail address. Did he move or change accounts?
18. She started sneezing the minute she entered the dusty attic. Does she have an allergy or an infection?
19. Will that be debit or credit? Is this about a checkbook or a charge card?
20. The black-tie event will honor the donors. Is this a formal or casual event?

BASIC MATH

Directions: Solve the problems.

1. 6 + 2 = ?
2. 7 + 6 = ?
3. 2 + 8 = ?
4. 7 + 8 = ?
5. 3 + 4 = ?
6. 5 + 7 = ?
7. 9 + 5 = ?
8. 8 + 3 = ?
9. 4 + 5 = ?
10. 8 + 9 = ?
11. 2 + 3 + 6 = ?
12. 7 + 1 + 5 = ?
13. 5 + 4 + 9 = ?
14. 8 + 8 + 4 = ?
15. 4 + 5 + 7 = ?
16. 1 + 7 + 2 = ?
17. 2 + 7 + 5 = ?
18. 4 + 8 + 6 = ?
19. 10 + 6 + 3 = ?
20. 5 + 4 + 3 = ?

Subtraction

Directions: Solve the problems.

1. 10 – 7 = ?
2. 14 – 9 = ?
3. 12 – 6 = ?
4. 9 – 5 = ?
5. 11 – 4 = ?
6. 18 – 5 = ?
7. 16 – 8 = ?
8. 13 – 4 = ?
9. 21 – 9 = ?
10. 17 – 7 = ?
11. 20 – 6 = ?
12. 24 – 8 = ?
13. 17 – 6 = ?
14. 20 – 7 = ?
15. 15 – 3 = ?
16. 11 – 2 = ?
17. 19 – 3 = ?
18. 14 – 2 = ?
19. 20 – 5 = ?
20. 13 – 7 = ?

Directions: Solve the problems.

1. $3 \times 3 = ?$
2. $7 \times 4 = ?$
3. $4 \times 5 = ?$
4. $3 \times 11 = ?$
5. $5 \times 5 = ?$
6. $5 \times 7 = ?$
7. $9 \times 9 = ?$
8. $7 \times 2 = ?$
9. $5 \times 8 = ?$
10. $6 \times 6 = ?$
11. $8 \times 9 = ?$
12. $4 \times 4 = ?$
13. $7 \times 7 = ?$
14. $8 \times 8 = ?$
15. $10 \times 6 = ?$
16. $3 \times 8 = ?$
17. $9 \times 2 = ?$
18. $5 \times 9 = ?$
19. $8 \times 7 = ?$
20. $7 \times 9 = ?$

Directions: Solve the problems.

1. $20 \div 10 = ?$
2. $15 \div 5 = ?$
3. $25 \div 5 = ?$
4. $16 \div 4 = ?$
5. $24 \div 3 = ?$
6. $21 \div 7 = ?$
7. $45 \div 5 = ?$
8. $30 \div 6 = ?$
9. $24 \div 2 = ?$
10. $70 \div 7 = ?$
11. $44 \div 4 = ?$
12. $14 \div 2 = ?$
13. $18 \div 3 = ?$
14. $12 \div 4 = ?$
15. $32 \div 8 = ?$
16. $63 \div 9 = ?$
17. $27 \div 3 = ?$
18. $72 \div 9 = ?$
19. $42 \div 7 = ?$
20. $30 \div 2 = ?$

Directions: Answer by telling if the items are equal or not.

1. Does $18 + 7 = 5 \times 5$?
2. Does $14 + 3 = 4 \times 4$?
3. Does $9 + 9 = 6 \times 3$?
4. Does $36 - 6 = 4 \times 8$?
5. Does $25 \times 3 = 12 \times 6$?
6. Does $20 + 4 = 3 + 2$?
7. Does $54 - 4 = 67 - 17$?
8. Does $48 + 6 = 7 \times 7$?
9. Does $3 + 9 = 7 + 7$?
10. Does $21 - 5 = 14 + 3$?
11. Does 20 pennies = 4 nickels?
12. Does 7 nickels = 3 dimes?
13. Does 2 quarters = 5 dimes?
14. Does 2 quarters = 12 nickels?
15. Does 8 nickels = 4 dimes?
16. Does 5 quarters = 3 half-dollars?
17. Does 2 dollars = 8 quarters?
18. Does 6 dimes + 4 nickels = 3 quarters + 1 dime?
19. Does 5 dimes = 5 nickels + 1 quarter?
20. Does 4 nickels + 1 quarter = 4 dimes?

Number Series

Directions: Give the next number in the sequence.

1. 2 3 4 ___
2. 10 20 30 ___
3. 8 10 12 ___
4. 20 25 30 ___
5. 59 53 47 ___
6. 17 15 13 ___
7. 120 110 100 ___
8. 84 88 92 ___
9. 25 45 65 ___
10. 3 9 15 ___
11. 70 69 68 ___
12. 45 40 35 ___
13. 11 22 33 ___
14. 8 16 24 ___
15. 100 97 94 ___
16. 75 66 57 ___
17. 89 82 75 ___
18. 3 6 9 ___
19. 13 20 27 ___
20. 66 62 58 ___

Directions: Follow the instructions.

1. Start with 10. Count by 2's to 20.
2. Start with 15. Count by 5's to 40.
3. Start with 6. Count by 3's to 21.
4. Start with 90. Count by 10 to 140.
5. Start with 32. Count by 4 to 52.
6. Start with 16. Count by 8 to 56.
7. Start with 7. Count by 7 to 42.
8. Start with 40. Count by 11 to 95.
9. Start with 30. Count by 6 to 60.
10. Start with 9. Count by 9 to 54.
11. Start with 53. Count by 2 to 63.
12. Start with 11. Count by 6 to 41.
13. Start with 14. Count by 3 to 29.
14. Start with 168. Count by 10 to 218.
15. Start with 85. Count by 4 to 105.
16. Start with 32. Count by 7 to 67.
17. Start with 97. Count by 5 to 122.
18. Start with 46. Count by 9 to 91.
19. Start with 2. Count by 11 to 57.
20. Start with 29. Count by 8 to 69.

Mental Math

Directions: Listen carefully as each problem is read, then figure the answer in your head.

1. Start with 10, add 6, divide by 2, add 4. What's the answer?
2. Start with 5, multiply by 3, add 3, subtract 1. What's the answer?
3. Start with 8, add 3, multiply by 3, subtract 3. What's the answer?
4. Start with 25, subtract 5, divide by 4, add 3. What's the answer?
5. Start with 12, add 2, add 8, divide by 2. What's the answer?
6. Start with 53, subtract 7, add 2, divide by 8. What's the answer?
7. Start with 71, add 4, add 25, divide by 10. What's the answer?
8. Start with 69, add 1, subtract 9, subtract 6. What's the answer?
9. Start with 4, multiply by 4, subtract 1, divide by 5. What's the answer?
10. Start with 100, subtract 7, subtract 9, subtract 4. What's the answer?
11. Start with 40, add 2, divide by 6, add 3. What's the answer?
12. Start with 38, add 7, subtract 5, divide by 5. What's the answer?
13. Start with 87, add 9, add 4, divide by 4. What's the answer?
14. Start with 2, multiply by 2, multiply by 4, add 4. What's the answer?
15. Start with 62, add 5, add 7, add 8. What's the answer?
16. Start with 9, add 9, divide by 3, subtract 2. What's the answer?
17. Start with 27, divide by 3, add 4, subtract 1. What's the answer?
18. Start with 6, divide by 3, multiply by 11, subtract 2. What's the answer?
19. Start with 3, add 12, multiply by 2, subtract 7. What's the answer?
20. Start with 7, add 6, subtract 5, multiply by 2. What's the answer?

Directions: Answer the questions.

1. How much money is 1 nickel and 2 dimes?
2. How much money is 2 quarters and 3 pennies?
3. How much money is 3 dimes and 7 pennies?
4. How much money is 2 quarters and 1 dime?
5. How much money is 3 nickels and 3 pennies?
6. How much money is 3 quarters and 1 nickel?
7. How much money is 1 quarter, 1 nickel, and 1 dime?
8. How much money is 1 half-dollar and 1 nickel?
9. How much money is 4 dimes and 2 pennies?
10. How much money is 6 pennies and 1 quarter?
11. How much money is 1 dollar, 5 dimes, 2 nickels, and 3 pennies?
12. How much money is 3 quarters, 2 dimes, and two $1 bills?
13. How much money is 10 dimes, 10 nickels, and 10 pennies?
14. How much money is 4 half-dollars, a dime, and a penny?
15. How much money is 7 nickels, 7 dimes, and 7 pennies?
16. How much money is 5 quarters, a nickel, and 4 pennies?
17. How much money is 8 quarters, a half-dollar, and 3 nickels?
18. How much money is a $50 bill, a quarter, and 5 nickels?
19. How much money is three $5 bills, two $10 bills, and seven $1 bills?
20. How much money is seven $1 bills, a $20 bill, and four $10 bills?

Coin Values

Receptive: Basic Math

Directions: Answer the questions by naming the correct coins.

1. What 2 coins would make 30¢?
2. What 3 coins would make 16¢?
3. What 2 coins would make 50¢?
4. What 5 coins would make 53¢?
5. What 4 coins would make 80¢?
6. What 5 coins would make 90¢?
7. What 4 coins would make 22¢?
8. What 5 coins would make 45¢?
9. What 4 coins would make 76¢?
10. What 8 coins would make 44¢?
11. What 4 coins would make 41¢?
12. What 2 coins would make 85¢?
13. What 6 coins would make $1.10?
14. What 6 coins would make 23¢?
15. What 5 coins would make 70¢?
16. What 8 coins would make 98¢?
17. What 7 coins would make 31¢?
18. What 6 coins would make $1.00?
19. What 7 coins would make 68¢?
20. What 8 coins would make $1.12?

Directions: Answer the questions with yes or no.

1. Does a cup of coffee usually cost more than $1?
2. Does a pair of gloves usually cost more than $100?
3. Does a twin mattress usually cost more than $1,500?
4. Does a pack of chewing gum usually cost more than $1?
5. Does an ice cream cone usually cost more than 75¢?
6. Does a dozen long-stemmed roses usually cost more than $20?
7. Does a DVD movie usually cost more than $50?
8. Does a gallon of milk usually cost more than 50¢?
9. Does a daily newspaper usually cost more than 5¢?
10. Does a new love seat usually cost more than $4,000?
11. Does a new car usually cost less than $5,000?
12. Does a piece of pizza usually cost less than $10?
13. Does a new pair of shoes usually cost less than $20?
14. Does a lobster dinner usually cost less than $10?
15. Does a night at a nice hotel usually cost less than $400?
16. Does it usually cost less than $100 to fly from New York to Los Angeles?
17. Does an average house in your area cost less than $150,000?
18. Does a gold necklace usually cost less than $10?
19. Does a fast-food hamburger usually cost less than $7?
20. Does a microwave oven usually cost less than $40?

Cost

Directions: Answer the questions with yes or no.

1. Does a pair of socks cost more than a pair of shoes?
2. Does a candy bar cost more than a salad bar?
3. Does a monthly magazine cost more than a daily newspaper?
4. Does a card table cost more than a deck of cards?
5. Does a Cadillac cost more than a computer?
6. Does a hammer cost more than a nail?
7. Does a plane ticket cost more than bus fare?
8. Does a babysitter cost more per hour than a lawyer?
9. Does gold usually cost more than silver?
10. Does a steak dinner cost more than a spaghetti dinner?
11. Does a glass of milk cost less than a glass of wine?
12. Does a lightbulb cost less than a lamp?
13. Does a bridal gown cost less than a nightgown?
14. Does a movie ticket cost less than a ticket to a Broadway play?
15. Does mailing a letter cost less than buying a large dog?
16. Does a bottle of shampoo cost less than a bottle of perfume?
17. Does buying a small house cost less than a camera?
18. Does a day at the beach cost less than a day at Sea World?
19. Does an umbrella cost less than a raincoat?
20. Does a big wedding cost less than a big funeral?

Directions: Figure out the answer in amount or in coins.

1. What type of change would you receive for a purchase of $3.90 from a $5 bill?
2. What type of change would you receive for a purchase of $36.50 from a $50 bill?
3. What type of change would you receive for a purchase of $15.74 from a $20 bill?
4. What type of change would you receive for a purchase of $.78 from a $1 bill?
5. What type of change would you receive for a purchase of $7.09 from a $10 bill?
6. What type of change would you receive for a purchase of $1.55 from a $5 bill?
7. What type of change would you receive for a purchase of $12.25 from a $20 bill?
8. What type of change would you receive for a purchase of $4.45 from a $5 bill?
9. What type of change would you receive for a purchase of $8.98 from a $10 bill?
10. What type of change would you receive for a purchase of $2.13 from a $5 bill?
11. Bob paid $4.08 for some stationery. He gave the clerk a $5 bill. What should he receive in change?
12. Jan paid $1.27 for a magazine. She gave the clerk $2. What should she receive in change?
13. Mary paid $14.35 for a vase. She gave the clerk a $20 bill. What should she receive in change?
14. Pat paid $27.46 for a shirt. He gave the clerk two $20 bills. What should he receive in change?
15. Jon paid $44.87 for a set of dishes. He gave the clerk three $20 bills. What should he receive in change?
16. Andy paid $7.65 for vitamins. He gave the clerk a $10 bill. What should he receive in change?
17. Ed paid $16.87 for a pizza. He gave the clerk a $20 bill. What should he receive in change?
18. Lisa paid $45.52 for a watch. She gave the clerk two $20 bills and a $10 bill. What should she receive in change?
19. Gene paid $28.23 for some books. He gave the clerk a $20 bill and a $10 bill. What should he receive in change?
20. Deb paid $78.60 for a small lamp. She gave the clerk two $50 bills. What should she receive in change?

Basic Conversions

Directions: Answer the questions.

1. How many inches in a foot?
2. How many days in a week?
3. How many nickels in a quarter?
4. How many minutes in an hour?
5. How many ounces in a cup?
6. How many cents in a dollar?
7. How many weeks in a year?
8. How many things in a dozen?
9. How many quarts in a gallon?
10. How many seconds in a minute?
11. How many feet in a yard?
12. How many pints in a quart?
13. How many hours in a day?
14. How many teaspoons in a tablespoon?
15. How many ounces in a pound?
16. How many months in a year?
17. How many years in a century?
18. How many dimes in a dollar?
19. How many days in a year?
20. How many inches in a yard?

Directions: Calculate the answer.

1. Change 2 pounds to ounces.
2. Change 6 feet to inches.
3. Change 80 nickels to dollars.
4. Change 3 gallons to quarts.
5. Change 120 minutes to hours.
6. Change 10 dollars to dimes.
7. Change 10 quarts to pints.
8. Change 180 seconds to minutes.
9. Change 36 things to pairs.
10. Change 5 years to months.
11. Change 6 weeks to days.
12. Change 5 dollars to quarters.
13. Change $\frac{12}{3}$ to a whole number.
14. Change 84 things to dozens.
15. Change 27 feet to yards.
16. Change 800 dollars to 20-dollar bills.
17. Change 96 hours to days.
18. Change 64 ounces to cups.
19. Change 4 yards to feet.
20. Change 2 pints to ounces.

More or Less

Directions: Answer the questions.

1. Is 3 yards more or less than 8 feet?
2. Is 3 dozen more or less than 30?
3. Is 3 quarts more or less than a gallon?
4. Is 14 minutes more or less than a ¼ hour?
5. Is the area in a square foot more or less than 150 square inches?
6. Is 6 ounces more or less than a ½ cup?
7. Is 17 inches more or less than a foot and a half?
8. Is 5 pints more or less than 5 cups?
9. Is 4 teaspoons more or less than 2 tablespoons?
10. Is 3 quarters more or less than 70 cents?
11. Is 5 gallons more or less than 10 quarts?
12. Is 100 seconds more or less than a minute and a half?
13. Is 16 feet more or less than 5 yards?
14. Is 30 hours more or less than a day and a half?
15. Is a ton more or less than 2,500 pounds?
16. Is 2 liters more or less than a quart?
17. Is 2 cups more or less than 2 pints?
18. Is a mile more or less than 5,000 feet?
19. Is 8 days more or less than a week?
20. Is a gross more or less than 150 items?

FUNCTIONAL MATERIAL

139 Coupons and Instructions ....*Coupons: What company is offering the coupon?*
Game instructions: What equipment is included with the game?

140 Recipes.......................................*Cookbook: Locate two recipes using onions.*
Recipe: How many will the recipe serve?

141 Medications................................*Over-the-counter medication: What is the maximum dosage per day?*
Prescription medication: Does it matter if you take this on an empty or full stomach?

142 Menus ....*Point out the most expensive item on the menu.*

143 Catalogs ....*Can you pay for an order when it is delivered?*

144 Magazines..................................*What is a feature that appears in every issue?*

145 Dictionary ....*What are three words starting with* ***phyt****?*

146 White Pages...............................*Find numbers for emergency, police, and fire.*

147 Yellow Pages ....*How many travel agencies are listed?*

148 Newspaper Sections 1................*Classified ads: How many pages of ads are there?*
Features / Local: Find an article about a local person.

149 Newspaper Sections 2................*Business: Name a person who is in the news and explain why.*
Stock: Give the date and the closing numbers for the Dow Jones, Standard & Poor's, and NASDAQ indicators.

150 Newspaper Sections 3................*Entertainment / Home: Who is the author of a feature story and what is it about?*
Sports: What is the major sports story?

151 Newspapers................................*Where are the comics located?*

152 Monthly Calendar.......................*On what day of the week does the next month start?*

153 Year Calendar ....*What is the name and date of a holiday that you do not celebrate?*

154 Local TV Guide..........................*When is the* Tonight Show *shown and on what channel?*

155 Cable TV Guide..........................*Name a movie, its release date, time, and star rating on the Comedy Channel.*

156 Internet Search...........................*www.msn.com Who is the second most popular* people search *for the week?*

157 Maps ....*Local map: Find and name an interstate highway.*
State map: What is the major east-west route through the state?

158 United States Map ....*Find and name the five Great Lakes.*

FUNCTIONAL MATERIAL

Directions: Use a coupon to answer the first set of questions and a set of game instructions for the second set.

Coupons

1. What company is offering the coupon?
2. What specific product and size is the coupon good for?
3. How much money would you save?
4. Where could you redeem the coupon?
5. Do you receive anything free?
6. Does the coupon have an expiration date?
7. How is the coupon to be used?
8. Are there any restrictions on the coupon?
9. Are there any times or places when the coupon is not valid?
10. What do you have to spend in order to save?

Instructions for a game

11. What equipment is included with the game?
12. Do you need any equipment not included in the package?
13. What are the least and the most number of players allowed?
14. If you lost or damaged a piece, where or who could you contact for a replacement?
15. What do you have to do to win? What is the goal?
16. How do you keep score? How do you keep track of who is ahead?
17. What skills do you need to play?
18. Do you need any specialized knowledge to play?
19. About how long will it take to complete a game?
20. How do you determine who goes first?

Directions: Use a general cookbook to answer the first set of questions and a recipe to answer the second set.

Cookbook

1. Locate two recipes using onions.
2. How many pie recipes are there?
3. If you had a lot of apples to use, how would you find recipes with apple as an ingredient?
4. If you want to plan a complete meal, are there menu selsctions? If so, where?
5. Is there information other than recipes? If so, what?
6. If you want a breakfast dish made with eggs and cheese, what is the fastest way to locate one?
7. Find a recipe with a foreign name.
8. What type of recipes is the book divided into?
9. Does each recipe tell you how long it takes to make, how many it serves, or the nutritional breakdown?
10. If you have a question about a recipe in the book, who would you contact?

Recipe

11. How many will the recipe serve?
12. How many different ingredients are needed?
13. Which ingredient will you need the least amount of?
14. Name the equipment you will need to complete the entire recipe.
15. About how long will it take from the time you start until the dish is ready to eat?
16. What would be the most difficult step?
17. Which ingredient could you probably leave out without hurting the final product?
18. What is another ingredient you could add to make it better?
19. When are two occasions you would serve this?
20. Could you buy this already made, and if so, where?

Directions: Use an over-the-counter medication to answer the first set of questions and a prescription medication to answer the second set.

Over-the-counter medication

1. What is the maximum dosage per day?
2. Is there a date after which the medication is not good?
3. What are the active ingredients?
4. Under what conditions should you not take this?
5. How is the product used (skin, mouth, etc.)?
6. Who is the manufacturer?
7. What is the maximum length of time you should stay on this product?
8. What types of ailments will the product help?
9. How should you store it?
10. What should you do in case of an overdose?

Prescription medication

11. Does it matter if you take this on an empty or full stomach?
12. What is the name of the place where the prescription was filled?
13. What is the phone number?
14. What is the name of the doctor who prescribed it?
15. How many times can it be refilled?
16. How many times a day do you take the medication?
17. What is the prescription number?
18. How many tablets or ounces are in the bottle?
19. How many days will this medication last?
20. What is the name of the medication?

Directions: Use the menu from a restaurant to answer the questions.

1. Point out the most expensive item on the menu.
2. How many different beverages could you order?
3. Choose a complete meal that you would enjoy. Figure out how much it would cost.
4. Are there restrictions on what time of day some items are served?
5. Can you buy anything for less than $1.50?
6. Is anything included with the main course?
7. What is the difference in price between the least and most expensive entrées on the menu?
8. Can you order a soup and salad? Is there a special price for salad with another item?
9. Can you make substitutions such as vegetables instead of potatoes?
10. How many desserts are listed, and what is their price range?
11. If you were hungry and in a hurry, what could you order that would be quick?
12. Could someone who is a vegetarian eat a full meal?
13. What type of food does the restaurant specialize in?
14. Can you order beer, wine, or a cocktail?
15. What is the difference in price between coffee, tea, and a soft drink?
16. Which salad dressings are available?
17. What is the least appealing thing to you on the menu?
18. What could you order as a full meal if you couldn't chew very well and needed soft foods?
19. What would be included in a medium-priced meal?
20. What would you order for a child about 10 years old?

Directions: Use a merchandise catalog (such as Lands' End, Pottery Barn, or Lillian Vernon) with an order form to answer the questions. You could also access a catalog over the Internet.

1. Can you pay for an order when it is delivered?
2. How do you place an order?
3. Find an item. How many colors does it come in?
4. Choose an item. Is there a different price if you buy more than one?
5. Choose an item. How would you identify it to a phone operator?
6. What questions might you have about the item which are **not** answered in the description?
7. If you ordered only one item costing $28, how much would the total bill be?
8. Do you have to pay shipping or handling charges? How are they calculated?
9. What can you do if you are not satisfied? What is the procedure to return a purchase?
10. What information do you need to know about the item to fill out the order blank?
11. Is there any way to get a discount on your purchases?
12. Do you have the option of ordering from a website?
13. Is there a toll-free number to call? If so, when can you call it, and what is the number?
14. Is there a choice of delivery methods? What is the fastest way to receive your order?
15. In which states is tax added to the order?
16. How many ways can you pay?
17. If you charge it, what information do you need to provide?
18. If you order over the phone, what information do you need to have ready?
19. Find an item that costs less than $25.
20. Make a list of at least four items that total just about $300.

Magazines

Directions: Use a magazine to answer the questions.

1. What is a feature that appears in every issue?
2. On what page is the table of contents and how is it arranged?
3. Find a story in the magazine that is featured on the cover. What page is it on?
4. How many full pages of advertising are in the first 25 pages of the magazine?
5. How much does the magazine cost?
6. Can you buy a subscription to the magazine, and if so, how much would it cost for a year?
7. How often is the magazine published?
8. Who is the editor of the magazine?
9. Can you submit articles or letters to the magazine? If so, how would you do it?
10. Name three celebrities who are pictured, quoted, or featured.
11. Do you enjoy this magazine? Why or why not?
12. Find the editor's column. Who wrote it and what is it about?
13. What three things could you learn from reading articles in this issue?
14. Could you order back issues of the magazine?
15. On what page does the first main article start?
16. Explain what the last feature in the magazine is about.
17. What feature would interest you the most?
18. Is there a preview of next month's articles?
19. How many articles are in the table of contents?
20. Does the cover give you any hint about the contents? How many teasers for articles are shown on the cover?

Directions: Use a dictionary to answer the questions.

1. What are three words starting with **phyt**?
2. What are two spellings of the word **ramekin**?
3. What are three definitions of **dragon**?
4. What does **steep** mean when used as a verb?
5. What is a two-word entry with **land** as the first word?
6. Is **whiffletree** one word or two?
7. How would you find out how high Niagara Falls is?
8. When was Marie Curie born?
9. What can the abbreviation **C.S.** stand for?
10. How many definitions does **short** have?
11. What is the last word in the dictionary? What does it mean?
12. What are three types of information given before the alphabetical listings?
13. Which letter has the least number of words?
14. What are the words just before and after **rendezvous**?
15. What is an **exegete**?
16. From what country does the word **rial** come?
17. What is a **candytuft**?
18. How many titles begin with **vice**?
19. Open to any page. What are the guide words on the page?
20. What does the last word that begins with **q** mean?

Directions: Use the white pages of a telephone book to answer the questions.

1. Find numbers for emergency, police, and fire.
2. What is on the inside back cover of the phone book?
3. Find someone whose last name begins with **L** and whose address is only a city.
4. How many columns of **Q** listings are there?
5. Locate information for the number to call if you have a question about your phone bill or service.
6. How many area codes are there for your state?
7. Is there a poison control number listed in the first few pages? If so, what is it?
8. What is the international access code to call overseas?
9. What is the country code for France and the city code for Paris?
10. Who published this phone book?
11. What does **res** mean when listed before an address?
12. How many listings are there for people with the last name of **Owens**?
13. On what page and in which column is your own listing?
14. Find a name (other than Smith or Jones) that fills more than one column.
15. What are the last two names in the book?
16. In the **A** listings, about how many listings are shown before the individual names start?
17. Is there a listing for someone whose last name is the same as your middle name?
18. What are the first and last **X** listings?
19. Find the listing for your local library.
20. Open to page 65. Go to the 14th name in the second column. What is the name and phone number of the listing?

Directions: Use the yellow pages of a telephone book to answer the questions.

1. How many travel agencies are listed?
2. If you needed your clothes dryer fixed, where would you look?
3. Find a physician specializing in dermatology and one in neurology.
4. How are restaurants listed and/or divided?
5. What can't you find in the yellow pages that you could in the white pages?
6. Where would you look to get rid of termites or carpenter ants?
7. Find a listing where you need to look under a second heading to find the information.
8. What are the listings under **Y**?
9. Name three types of information that appear before the alphabetical listings.
10. What are two listings between **Caterers** and **Chiropractors**?
11. What is the number of the third florist listed?
12. What different headings could you check if you wanted to buy a diamond?
13. Look up the listing for furniture. How many places are within 10 miles of your home?
14. Locate a place where you could rent tables, chairs, and tablecloths.
15. Find three headings with only one listing under each.
16. What headings start with the word *security*?
17. On what page is a listing for an interpreter? What is the name of the heading?
18. Name two headings where you could find computers.
19. Are there more listings for insurance or mortgage companies?
20. Are there more listings for condominiums or apartments?

Newspaper Sections 1

Directions: Use the classified ads section of a newspaper to answer the first 10 questions and the features or local section for the final 10 questions.

Classified Ads

1. How many pages or columns of ads are there? Answer whichever is less.
2. What is the most unusual thing in the Lost and Found section?
3. What is the ad on the third page, second column, and fourth up from the bottom?
4. What ads are listed for a recent year Corvette?
5. What kind of puppies could you take home today?
6. What is the first job offering you see in sales? Where is it? What qualifications do you need?
7. If you were an engineer, could you find any jobs available in that field?
8. What is an intriguing ad under Dating Services or Personal Ads?
9. What is the phone number and specialty of the second Legal Services listing?
10. Pick an apartment rental and give the information about it.

Features or Local Section

11. Find an article about a local person and explain why the person is newsworthy.
12. Find an event happening in your community and give the details.
13. Turn to the third page and the second column. What article do you find there?
14. Find a full- or half-page ad. What is the product and what is the pitch?
15. What is the most interesting article to you in this section?
16. Look for a restaurant review or article and give a summary of the information.
17. What is a feature in this section that appears at least weekly?
18. Is there an article about your hometown? What is it about?
19. Look for information about a store and tell why it was mentioned.
20. Pick a short article and tell what it is about.

Directions: Use the business section of a newspaper to answer the first 10 questions and the stock pages for the final 10 questions.

Business Section

1. Name a person who is in the news and explain why.
2. What is the message of a major ad in this section?
3. Look for a column written by an individual. Explain its main message.
4. Find a story about a company in financial trouble or that is claiming bankruptcy.
5. What are the headlines in this section?
6. Find a paragraph about a company and explain why it is newsworthy.
7. Find some information about an overseas company.
8. Look for an article about a retail store. What is the store and why is it written up?
9. Find a story that begins on the front page and continues on another page.
10. Look at the caption under a picture and explain what it is about.

Stock Pages

11. Give the date and the closing numbers for the Dow Jones, Standard & Poor's, and NASDAQ indicators.
12. What are the top five most active stocks?
13. What is the U.S. dollar worth in Canada?
14. What is the closing price of gold (COMX)?
15. What stock is the biggest loser for the day?
16. What are two statistics given for Kellogg stock?
17. How many stocks begin with the letter *Q*?
18. Name the types of Fidelity mutual funds.
19. What is the closing price and the change for the LifeGro Vanguard Fund?
20. Which American Fund shows the highest price change?

Newspaper Sections 3

Directions: Use the entertainment / home section of a newspaper to answer the first 10 questions and the sports section for the final 10 questions.

Entertainment / Home section

1. Who is the author of a feature story and what is it about?
2. Find an ad for a first-run movie and name its producer and rating.
3. Find an article about a product. What is the product used for and is it recommended?
4. What is a concert that is coming to your area and how much are tickets?
5. What is an event taking place near your home this weekend?
6. Give the names of any recipes or other food reviews listed in the section.
7. What is a TV show that is singled out with some extra information about it?
8. What is the smallest bit of information that is on the second page?
9. What are the teaser headlines at the very top of the page?
10. In the Movie Guide, find the theater that has the most number of screens.

Sports section

11. What is the major sports story?
12. Name a columnist and the subject of the column.
13. What sport, if any, has a complete page devoted to it?
14. Name an athlete in the news.
15. Name two major league teams that lost. What was the sport and who were the teams?
16. Are any sports teams in playoff games? If so, what are they?
17. Is there an ad for some type of athletic equipment? What is the sale price?
18. Find a local sports story. Explain what it is about.
19. Where are the college scores listed and for what sport(s)?
20. Find a quote by a coach about why a game was won or lost.

Directions: Use a whole newspaper to answer the questions.

1. Where are the comics located?
2. How many sections are in the paper? What are their titles?
3. What is the lead story? Are there other stories related to it?
4. What features are always on the last page?
5. Name three features that are in every newspaper.
6. Locate a major story. Tell where it took place and who wrote it.
7. What are the latest winning lottery numbers in a daily game?
8. How would you place an ad in this paper?
9. Find Microsoft stock in the listings. Give its sale price and its daily high and low prices.
10. Name each of the sections in the paper.
11. Who is the publisher of the paper?
12. If you wanted to write a letter to the editor, where would you send it?
13. Find a column by someone who writes a regular feature. Explain what he or she writes about.
14. What is something your horoscope says?
15. Name something that appears on the inside of the front page.
16. Name the first and last persons listed in the death notices.
17. Name something that is included in the Sunday edition of this paper that is not included during the week.
18. What are the expected low and high temperatures for the day?
19. What is found on the editorial page besides an editorial?
20. Is there a crossword puzzle in the paper? What is the definition for 10 down?

Monthly Calendar

Directions: Use a monthly calendar to answer the questions.

1. On what day of the week does the next month start?
2. What day of the week is the 16th?
3. What will the date be on the third Thursday of the month?
4. How many Sundays are in the month?
5. What are the dates of all the Tuesdays?
6. What day does the last day of the month fall on?
7. What is the date three weeks from the first Friday of the month?
8. What are the dates of the last full weekend in the month?
9. If the second of the month were a Wednesday, what day would the 18th be?
10. What is the date of the Monday following the second Saturday?
11. How many Wednesdays are in the month?
12. What is the day and date of two weeks from the 3rd?
13. How many Saturdays are odd numbers?
14. What date is the second Saturday after the 4th?
15. You are hosting a party on the 20th and want your carpet cleaned. The company can only come on a Wednesday or a Monday. What date will you have them come?
16. You are going out of town on the first Friday of the month and will return four days later. What dates will you be gone?
17. You need to complete a report by the last Thursday of the month. You need five days to write the report. When should you start writing?
18. How many even-numbered weekend dates are there?
19. Assume it is the 24th of the month. What day of the week is two weeks before that?
20. What, if any, special days does this month show?

Directions: You will need a calendar that shows all the days of the year to answer the questions.

1. What is the name and date of a holiday that you do not celebrate?
2. What is the ninety-ninth day of the year?
3. How many weeks are between Memorial Day and Independence Day?
4. What is the date of the fourth day of the fourth week of the fourth month?
5. On what date could you say "only 35 more shopping days until Christmas"?
6. What months start on Friday and have 30 days?
7. What are the dates of all the Tuesdays in November?
8. How many months have the first of the month on a Sunday?
9. How many days are between your birthday and a major holiday?
10. What date is 21 days past Valentine's Day?
11. How many months have 31 days?
12. How many days apart are March 24 and April 6?
13. How many holidays are shown? How many are on a Monday or a Friday?
14. On what day of the week is June 23?
15. Find your birthday. How many weeks into the year is it?
16. You place an order on September 17 and are told it will be delivered in 10 working days. On what day should you expect it?
17. How many days are between Thanksgiving and Christmas?
18. How many weekdays are in February?
19. How many Mondays are on the 20th of the months?
20. If you make an appointment on April 3 for June 15, how many weeks ahead will you be making it?

Directions: Use a weekly TV guide to answer the questions.

1. When is the *Tonight Show* shown and on what channel?
2. Find a show that starts between 7:30 and 8:30 on Tuesday evening.
3. How many programs start at 4:30 P.M. on Wednesday?
4. How many different news shows are listed between 5:00 and 7:30 P.M.?
5. How can you tell if the show is a rerun or a new episode?
6. How many days does the guide cover?
7. For how long a time period is *The Today Show* on each day?
8. What is a show you could see on cable but not on the regular networks?
9. Name three shows for children shown weekday mornings between 7:30 and 11:30.
10. How can you tell if a program is a movie?
11. Name a prime-time game show and when it is televised.
12. Which day lists more sporting events than any other?
13. Name a PBS station shown on Sunday afternoon between 3:00 and 4:00.
14. What shows are on NBC between 1:00 and 3:00 A.M. during the week?
15. Name a game show and tell when it is seen.
16. Name three soap operas and tell when they are shown.
17. What are the choices at 9:00 Thursday evening on ABC, NBC, and CBS?
18. On how many channels can you watch the news at 11:00 P.M.?
19. Name a show that is recommended and is listed in the front of the guide.
20. How many different shows could you watch Monday evening between 9:00 and 10:00?

Directions: You will need a cable TV grid for one day for this exercise. Use the guide to answer the questions.

1. Name a movie, its release date, time, and star rating on the Comedy Channel.
2. Name a series on the BRAVO station.
3. What show is on the Food Channel at 8:00 P.M. weekdays?
4. What is a syndicated sitcom that is shown on *Nick at Nite*?
5. Name two news show hosts on CNN.
6. Find a movie that starts at 6:00 P.M. What is the network, channel, movie, and star?
7. Name a station that shows repeats of *Friends*.
8. How many HBO channels are there?
9. How many movies start at 8:00 P.M. on regular (not premium) cable channels?
10. What show might appeal to you on the Food Channel?
11. What sport has a channel all to itself?
12. How many different shows are shown between 6:00 and 11:00 P.M. on MTV?
13. How many cable channels start with the letter *T*?
14. Are there any channels that broadcast the same show at 8:00 and 11:00? What are they?
15. Name two shows on HGTV that you might watch.
16. If you wanted to watch sports commentaries, what stations would you check?
17. How many cable channels are listed in your guide?
18. What show comes on at 10:30 on TBS?
19. Find two game shows and the times they are shown.
20. When is the program *Hardball* and on what network is it shown?

Internet Search

Directions: Use a computer with Internet capabilities for this exercise. Visit the website given for the first 10 questions; for the final ten, use a search engine to answer the questions.

1. www.msn.com Who is the second most popular *people search* for the week?
2. www.akc.org Find the spotlighted breed of the month and two facts about it.
3. www.guinnessworldrecords.com What is the longest recorded time for balancing on one foot?
4. www.pgatour.com Go to *players* and find out how many events Tiger Woods has played this year and what his average score is.
5. www.foodnetwork.com What is the recipe of the day from Paula Deen?
6. www.quotationspage.com What is the third quotation by Benjamin Franklin?
7. www.800padutch.com What is the answer to the third most frequently asked question about the Amish?
8. www.rd.com How do you submit a joke and how much will you be paid if your joke is published in the magazine?
9. www.wendys.com How many calories and sodium does a classic double burger with cheese have?
10. www.elvis.com How much is a Graceland Platinum Tour ticket for one adult in a group?
11. Who are the Supreme Court justices? Who has served the longest?
12. What is Engelbert Humperdinck's real name?
13. What does IKEA stand for?
14. When did Walt Disney die and what was his cause of death?
15. Why can chocolate be poisonous to dogs?
16. What is the cheapest fare you can find to fly tomorrow from Detroit to Baltimore?
17. Search for your full name on the web. What do you find?
18. Find a picture crossword puzzle. Print it and complete it.
19. What are the *Farmer's Almanac* weather predictions for this month in your area?
20. What is the definition of aphasia according to the National Aphasia Association?

Directions: Use a map of local places to answer the first 10 questions and a map of the United States to answer the final 10 questions.

Local map

1. Find and name an interstate highway.
2. Find two streets that begin with *F*. What are they?
3. Name something at the intersection of *B-4*.
4. Locate a body of water in the index, then find it on the map.
5. Find your home and show the route you take to a store where you shop.
6. Find and name a county on the map.
7. How many miles does a one-inch line reflect?
8. Locate a town in small print and the name of a larger town close to it. In what direction is the second place from the first?
9. Locate an intersection of two main roads. What are their names?
10. Find and name a park, historical site, or school.

State map

11. What is the major east-west route through the state?
12. Using a legend, about how far do you live from the capital?
13. What towns are directly north, south, east, and west of your hometown?
14. Name a town in your state that is on the border of another state.
15. Find two cities in two parts of the state. Map a route between them.
16. Find three towns beginning with the letter *C*.
17. Find an airport. What is its official name?
18. Name any cities that have an inset map to show more detail.
19. What is the name of the largest body of water within the state?
20. Measure one inch in any direction from your hometown and name two places at that mark.

Directions: Use a map of the United States that shows major highways to answer the questions.

1. Find and name the five Great Lakes.
2. How many states touch Oklahoma? Name them.
3. If you drive from Philadelphia to Miami, what states will you go through?
4. What places surround Maine?
5. What are two towns / cities in Alaska besides Juneau and Anchorage?
6. Name all the states north and east of Pennsylvania.
7. Locate the Gulf of Mexico. Name two cities in different states that are on the gulf.
8. How many states west of Michigan share a border with Canada?
9. If you travel from Texas to Florida, what states will you go through?
10. Name the states from North Dakota south to Mexico.
11. What interstate highway goes through Albuquerque, Knoxville, and Oklahoma City?
12. What interstate highway would you take from Denver to Chicago?
13. Follow Interstate 35 south from Duluth. Where does it end?
14. Name a town on Cape Cod.
15. Name two mountain ranges west of the Mississippi.
16. What is the closest city across the Canadian border from Seattle?
17. What city is the most southern in the U.S. and what is the most northern (not including Alaska)?
18. What one interstate could take you from Bangor, Maine, to Miami, Florida?
19. Name four states that come together at one point.
20. What one interstate could you take from Sacramento, California, to New York City?

PARAGRAPHS

Note: Only one comprehension question is shown per exercise.

161 Multiple Clues ....*It is an animal. It has a flat tail. It builds dams. Is it a beaver or a porcupine?*

163 Infer Situations ....*The lights dimmed. The music began. The curtain rose. What is the situation?*

165 Basic Facts.................................*Chili powder is actually a combination of several spices including chili peppers, cloves, garlic, cumin, and oregano. The amount of each can differ by recipe and brand. Is there garlic in chili?*

167 Basic Sequential Information ....*She went in the house. She put the grocery bag on the chair. She put her purse down and then got the mail. What did she do last?*

169 Basic Directions.........................*Take one tablet in the morning on an empty stomach either one hour before or two to three hours after a meal unless otherwise directed by your doctor. How many tablets are taken a day?*

171 Basic Conversation.....................*We are expecting about 100 walkers. All the volunteers have checked in and are going to their posts. The water bottles and T-shirts are being unloaded now. What is the event?*

173 Basic Everyday Information ....*John left work at 7:30. He stopped and got a paper. He drove two more miles and picked up Paul, his carpool buddy. Who is the passenger?*

175 Basic Messages...........................*This is Barnes & Noble calling. Your special book order has arrived. The book is* Small Ways to Reduce Big Stress. *You can pick it up at the main desk any time after 5:00 today. When can you pick it up?*

177 Basic Instructions ....*An easy way to clean a blender is to fill it about halfway with water. Add a few drops of liquid dish soap. Cover the blender and turn it on medium for about a minute. What do you add to the water?*

180 Inconsistencies...........................*It was a hot, humid day. The air conditioner was working full-time to keep the house somewhat cool. Some relief from the heat came from closing the blinds to keep the sun out and opening the windows to bring in a breeze. What does not make sense in the story?*

182 Everyday Information................*The mail was mostly ads, but it had a few surprises. An unexpected dividend check came from a stock split as well as an invitation to a surprise 50th birthday party. The rest of the mail was bills, a* Consumers Report *magazine, and a new VISA card. Why was there a check in the mail?*

185 Multiple Ideas............................*Baby Wipes have a number of uses. 1) They are great for shining up faucets and dashboards in cars. 2) They can clean and polish leather shoes. 3) They can be used to blot up stains that are still wet. What was the second use?*

189 Messages....................................*I will meet you at Bud's Beefsteak Tavern after work on Friday. The Tavern used to be Chang's Chinese and is in the Woodland Square Strip mall. The mall is on the west side of Woodward near Lincoln. In what mall is it located?*

192 Sequential Information ....*The first gallery you will pass through has paintings by American women. The next room has Amish quilts hanging on the walls. The last room to your left has antique jewelry and the room beyond that on the right has a replica of a working blacksmith shop. What is the third exhibit you will pass?*

196 Facts...*In the first three months of their lives, baby pelicans eat about 150 pounds of fish. The baby birds need extra fat to survive during the time they are learning to fish for their own food. When the young birds leave the nest at about five weeks of age, they are often heavier than their parents. Why do the birds need fat?*

201 Conversations ....***A:*** *Do you come here often?* ***B:*** *No, it's my first time. I came with a friend who is a regular.* ***A:*** *Can I buy you a drink?* ***B:*** *No thanks, we're waiting for a table and we could be called any minute. Where does this take place?*

204 Lists..*This is a list of common things with uncommon names. A heeltap is the tiny bit of liquid left in a glass after you have finished drinking. The grumbling sound of an upset stomach is called wamble. The holder that is put around paper cups that contain hot liquids is a zarf. The lunula is the small white half-moon part of your nails. What is wamble?*

Directions: Listen to the sentences, and then choose the correct answer from the choices.

1. It is an animal. It has a flat tail. It builds dams.
   Is it a beaver or a porcupine?
2. It is used to regulate temperature. It runs on gas, electricity, or oil. It provides heat.
   Is it an air conditioner or a furnace?
3. It is used in the office and the home. It holds papers together. It is metal.
   Is it a staple or scissors?
4. It is used to repair things. It is sticky. It comes on a roll.
   Is it masking tape or glue?
5. It is a large state. It borders on water. It has mostly warm and hot weather.
   Is it Alaska or Texas?
6. It is used in sewing. It has a sharp point. It is threaded.
   Is it a needle or a pin?
7. It is a dish. It is round. It is used under a cup.
   Is it a saucer or a bowl?
8. It is a food. It can be used on hamburgers. It is yellow.
   Is it ketchup or mustard?
9. It is a car. It is sporty. The top can be lowered.
   Is it a convertible or a minivan?
10. It is a vegetable. It can be green or red. It is used to make coleslaw.
    Is it broccoli or cabbage?
11. It is a bird. It can be taught words. It can be kept as a pet.
    Is it a parrot or a robin?
12. It is used in a bathroom. It is a cleaning agent. It is used on hair.
    Is it soap or shampoo?
13. It comes in many colors. It is used on a bed. It is usually made of cotton.
    Is it a sheet or a pillow?
14. It is used in salad dressings. It can be flavored. It is sour.
    Is it vinegar or oil?
15. It shows the time. It makes noise. It is supposed to wake you.
    Is it a stopwatch or a clock radio?

16. It is placed on the floor. It can be plain or patterned. It is put in front of a door.
    Is it a welcome mat or a carpet?

17. It is a citrus fruit. It is not sweet. It can be added to tea for flavor.
    Is it a lemon or an orange?

18. It is used on a bulletin board. It has a head. It can be pushed in with your finger.
    Is it a thumbtack or a nail?

19. It can be a liquid, gel, or solid. It is used to cover body odor. It is used under the arms.
    Is it perfume or deodorant?

20. They are worn inside. They are for the feet. They are found next to beds.
    Are they sneakers or slippers?

Directions: Identify the event that is described.

What is the situation being described?

1. The lights dimmed. The music began. The curtain rose.
2. She heard the doorbell and jumped. She made a final check in the mirror. She took a deep breath, put her hand on the knob, smiled widely, and opened the door.
3. About 20 people are walking in a line in front of a clinic. They are carrying signs and shouting to the people and cars passing by. Two policemen are watching from their squad car.
4. You could see a white streak of smoke in the sky. Seconds later, a loud but distant roar could be heard.
5. Bill moved a red disk diagonally one square. Tom took a black disk, lifted it over the red one, and then took the red disk.
6. He entered the four-digit code and waited for the next question on the screen. He pushed the keys, waited, and then took money from the slot.
7. The woman wearing dark glasses was holding the harness of the large dog. As they approached a curb, the dog stopped.
8. All preparation was complete. All systems checked. Begin countdown. Ten, nine, eight, seven, six, five, four, three, two, one, ignition, lift-off.
9. The man wore a stocking over his head and carried a small knife in his hand. He crouched behind a bush, waiting for the last light in the house to go out.
10. Skewers of meat, onions, peppers, and tomatoes were placed on a rack over the hot coals.
11. The car slowed. The driver took a quarter and tossed it into a bin. A green light flashed, and a gate went up.
12. He could feel his heart pounding in his chest. His arms and legs felt limp, and he was breathing very fast.
13. A piece of paper is placed face-down on the glass. The lid is closed, and a button is pushed. A few seconds later another sheet with the same markings as the first one appears.
14. The girl took her seat at the bench. She leaned the book against the holder and opened it to page 6. She positioned her fingers on the keys and feet on the pedals.
15. The cat's back was arched. Its tail was twitching and its fur was standing straight up on end.

16. He raced toward the net and brought his racket back. It connected with the ball, which sailed across the net to the back court where the volley was returned.

17. The girl slid the window open and handed the sack to the man in the car. The man paid the girl $3.84. She said, "Have a nice day," and slid the window shut.

18. The stage had eight large amplifiers and speakers on stands. Four microphones were positioned in the front. Drums were on a platform at the rear.

19. Devastation was everywhere. Roofs were ripped off buildings; windows were blown out. Debris was spread all over the yards and streets.

20. One man approached another in a dark alley. The first one said, "Have you got it?" The other said, "Five kilos. Where's the cash?"

Directions: Listen to the information and answer the questions.

1. Chili powder is actually a combination of several spices including chili peppers, cloves, garlic, cumin, and oregano. The amount of each can differ by recipe and brand.
   Is chili powder a combination of two spices? Is there garlic in chili powder?

2. The Shiba Inu is a Japanese dog that looks like a small fox.
   Is the dog Chinese? Does it look like a fox?

3. There is more calcium in your body than any other mineral. Calcium is found in the bones and teeth.
   Is calcium a mineral? Is there calcium in your teeth?

4. An official drop of water weighs almost a gram. There are 60 drops of water in one teaspoon.
   Does a drop of water weigh more than a gram? Can 50 drops fit in one teaspoon?

5. The original game of Monopoly was manufactured by Parker Brothers. There is more Monopoly money produced each year than money printed by the government.
   Is Monopoly still produced? Does Parker Brothers print real money?

6. By definition, a desert receives less than 10 inches of rain a year. All of the continents except Europe have deserts.
   Can a desert get eight inches of rain a year? Do all the continents have deserts?

7. Although we think of the eggplant as a vegetable, it is really a fruit. It is related to the tomato, which is another fruit.
   Is an eggplant a vegetable? Is a tomato a vegetable?

8. Bats have the best hearing of any land animal. They send out sound waves. When the waves hit objects, an echo comes back to the bat.
   Do bats hear like humans? Do bats hear well?

9. The Corn Palace in Mitchell, South Dakota, is decorated with kernels of corn and other parts of the corn plant. It is also known as the "world's largest bird feeder."
   Is the palace in North Dakota? Do birds like the Palace?

10. A puggle is a mixed-breed dog that mates a beagle and a pug. The resulting dog can have fewer breathing problems than a pug and the sweet temperament of a beagle.
    Would a puggle make a good family pet? Is a puggle a cross between a poodle and a beagle?

11. The first jigsaw puzzle was developed in 1760 by a teacher who glued a map to a piece of wood and cut the countries apart on their boundary lines.
    Did the man invent crossword puzzles? Was the first puzzle on wood?

12. Have you ever noticed how many earthworms you see during a rain? This is because earthworms breathe through their skin, and would drown if they stayed in the wet mud.
    Do earthworms live in the ground? Can earthworms die in mud?

13. Early Egyptians did not like hair. Men and women shaved their scalps and wore wigs.
    Did the Egyptians shave their heads? Did only the men wear wigs?

14. The inventor of Velcro was Swiss. He got his inspiration when some burrs stuck to his jacket after he took a walk in the woods.
    Did an American develop Velcro? Do burrs stick to clothing?

15. Lipstick began from a superstition. It was believed that a red circle around the mouth kept the soul inside the body and the devil outside.
    Was lipstick always used for beauty? Was lipstick thought to keep the devil away?

16. The original cowboy boots had heels so they wouldn't slip through the stirrups. Leather stitching on the boots kept them from wrinkling.
    Do the heels on cowboy boots serve a purpose? Do the boots have stitching on them?

17. According to statistics, men can read smaller print than women can. But women can hear better than men.
    Whose hearing is better? Who can read smaller print?

18. Hair on your head grows about five inches a year. For some reason, dark hair grows faster than light-colored hair.
    Does light hair grow faster than dark hair? Does hair grow more than two inches a year?

19. In major-league baseball, the bases are exactly 90 feet apart. Each base must be 15 inches square.
    Are there 100 feet between the bases? Are the bases longer than a foot?

20. Garlic is also known as the "stinking rose." It can help keep fleas and mosquitoes away from pets and humans.
    Can garlic help protect you from bites? Do fleas like garlic?

Directions: Listen to the information and answer the questions.

1. She went in the house. She put the grocery bag on the chair. She put her purse down and then got the mail.
   What did she do when she got in the house? What did she do last?

2. He hauled the cooler into the sailboat. He checked to see how many life jackets were on board. He began to take the covers off the seats.
   What did he bring into the boat? What did he check?

3. His first time at bat he hit a double. The second time he struck out. Then he walked on four balls.
   Which was his worst time at bat? Did he have a base hit?

4. Mom picked up her daughter at 3:30. She dropped her off at the door to go sign in. Meantime, Mom went to park. The daughter was third on the list to get an allergy shot.
   What happened before she parked? Why did she pick up her daughter?

5. She put the water in a pot to boil. She turned on the oven to heat the bread. She got out a box of frozen peas.
   What did she do first? What did she do last?

6. One thing after another went wrong all day. First, she dropped a plate and it broke. Then she spilled cereal on the floor. And now she can't find her glasses.
   What did she spill? What was the first thing that went wrong?

7. He was not very excited about painting, but he put down the drop cloths. He checked the refrigerator and made himself a ham sandwich. He went to the basement to get the paint roller and pan.
   What did he do before he ate? Where was the equipment?

8. The baby grabbed for the stuffed animal. Then she laughed when she was tickled. She let out a yell when her mother picked her up.
   Why did she laugh? What did the baby do first?

9. First, he checked his email. Then he got himself a big mug of coffee. Then he listened to his phone messages.
   What did he do before he got coffee? What was the last thing he did?

10. He turned on the grill. He brought out a platter of hamburgers and put it on the table by the grill. He went back in the house to get some seasoned salt.
    What did he forget on his first trip? Is it a gas or charcoal grill?

11. The power went off at 2:34 A.M. I got my flashlight from the nightstand by the bed. I opened the door to check outside and smelled a skunk. By the time I got back in the bedroom, the power had come back on.
    About how long was the power out? What happened after the speaker got a flashlight?

12. She explained that the historical walking tour would cover about four blocks. She handed out brochures and a coupon to the science museum. She said many of the buildings they would see date back to the eighteenth century.
    What was the first thing she explained? What did she hand out?

13. She really needed change. She looked in the bottom of her purse. She looked on top of the dresser and in the pockets of all her jackets. Then she looked in the armrest and on the floor of the car.
    What was she looking for? Where was the third place she looked?

14. I received seven ads in the door from companies who want to fertilize the lawn. I called Beautiful Green but their prices were too high. Then last week I left a message at Lovely Lawns, but no one has called me back.
    Who did you contact first? Who has not returned your calls?

15. She called to reserve a table for four on Saturday. She called back to ask if they could supply a birthday cake. Then she called to add four more people to the table.
    Why did she call back the first time? Why did she call the last time?

16. He put three quarters in the parking meter, then he went into Kinko's. He had to color copy the 15-page report, then he laminated four charts.
    What did he have to copy? What did he do before he went into the store?

17. First cross the bridge over the Rouge River. Then you will pass a fire station on your left. When you get to the traffic light, turn right.
    What will you see on your left? When do you turn right?

18. They will fly to Orlando for two days at Universal Studios. Then they will rent a car and drive to Cape Canaveral. There they will tour the Space Center and spend the night. The next day they will board the Disney Cruise Ship.
    What is the least number of days they will be on land in Florida? Where will they visit just before taking a cruise?

19. When he went to get the paper, he found the trash can on its side with its contents all over. Then he noticed scratch marks on the garage door. After he found paw prints in the mud, he knew it must have been a hungry raccoon.
    What was the first clue that something was wrong? What was the deciding factor as to what caused the can to tip?

20. The shopping center was open during construction, but customers had to go in through the back entrance. Parking was only allowed behind the stores. People were supposed to wait for a shuttle to take them around to the front entrances. At that point, they had to go through a covered walkway that led directly into a store.
    What did you do after you parked? Why wasn't parking allowed in the usual spots?

Directions: Listen to the information and answer the questions.

1. Take one tablet in the morning on an empty stomach either one hour before or two to three hours after a meal unless otherwise directed by your doctor.
   How many tablets are taken a day? Can you take this with food?

2. Machine wash in warm water, gentle cycle. Do not bleach. Line dry or tumble on low.
   Where would you see this information? Can you put this piece in the regular cycle?

3. Explanation of benefits. This is not a bill. This statement reports a claim was recently processed for you. Please review the claim for accurate information. You have met your deductible for the year.
   Where would you read this? How much do you owe?

4. Under penalty of law this tag may not be removed except by the consumer. Certification is made by the manufacturer that the materials in this article are described in accordance with the law.
   Where would you find this information? Who cannot remove the tag?

5. Deal out five cards to each player. Stack the rest of the cards facedown in the center of the playing field. Turn over the first card.
   What are the directions for? How many cards do you deal out?

6. Do not run on deck. No food or beverage past this point. Running, rough play, and excessive noise are forbidden. No swimming in diving area.
   Where would you see this information? Who is the information mostly meant for?

7. In case there is a loss of air pressure, mask will drop down. Grasp mask and pull toward you. Place the mask over your nose and mouth. Adjust the elastic band and breathe normally. Secure the mask over your own face before helping others.
   What are the directions for? How does the mask stay on?

8. Press 1 to hear business hours. Press 2 if you have billing questions. Press 3 if you have an emergency. Press 4 to speak with an actual person. Our lines are currently busy. Please hold for the next available representative.
   Where would you hear this information? Why would you push number 3?

9. Thirty-six animals are hidden in the grid. Look horizontally, vertically, and diagonally. Letters can be found running forward or backward but always in a straight line. Circle each word as you find it.
   What are the directions for? How can the words be hidden?

10. Enter your PIN number, then press here. Do you want a deposit or withdrawal? Do you want a withdrawal from your checking or savings account? What amount do you wish to withdraw?
    What are the directions for? What information must you know for this service?

11. The information contained in this transmission is privileged and confidential. It is intended only for the use of the individual or entity named above. If you have received this communication in error, please notify us immediately by telephone at the number listed above.
    What kind of transmission is it? What should you do if this was sent to the wrong place?

12. For normal washing conditions, fill cup to line 1 for medium loads and line 2 for large loads. Add liquid as washer fills with water. Continue washing as usual.
    What product are the directions for? How much would you use if you had a small load?

13. Preheat oven to 425°. Remove frozen loaf from plastic bag and place on an ungreased baking sheet or wrap it in aluminum foil. When the temperature is reached, place the loaf on the middle shelf of oven. Heat 10 to 15 minutes until heated through.
    What product are the directions for? Where should it be placed in the oven?

14. No dogs allowed. No glass bottles, alcoholic beverages, or other controlled substances permitted. No motorized vehicles of any kind. Organized groups of more than 12 must apply for a permit. No fires of any kind are permitted.
    Where would you see this information? What types of beverages are allowed?

15. To protect against electric shock, do not immerse cord, plug, or base in water or any other liquid. Plug in appliance. Move switch to low or high position as desired. Hold appliance at least 12 inches from head and move back and forth over wet areas. Do not point appliance at face.
    What product are the directions for? How should you hold the appliance?

16. Please pay minimum payment due. Finance charges accrue from the date it is added to your daily balance until payment in full is received on your account.
    Where would you see this information? When you should you pay this?

17. Put ½ to 1 inch of pea gravel in the bottom of the container. Mix half peat moss with half potting soil, and fill the container about two-thirds full. Arrange plants as you want, remembering to put trailing plants toward the outside of the container and tall plants in the middle.
    What are the directions for? What do you mix into the container?

18. Shake bottle well. Before using, wipe up excess material or stain from the carpet. Then thoroughly soak all stained areas with the product. Wait five minutes, then blot with a white absorbent cloth or paper towel until all stains have been removed. Repeat application if necessary.
    What product are the directions for? What do you do after five minutes?

19. In addition to Form 1099, file Form 1099-MISC for miscellaneous income. This includes rent or royalty payments, prizes and awards that are not for services, such as winnings on TV or radio shows. This also includes fish purchases paid in cash for resale.
    Where would you find these instructions? If you won a trip or a door prize, would you need this form?

20. Good for 75 cents off your next purchase. Must be used for large or economy size. Cannot be combined with any other offer. Expires December 2008.
    Where would you find this information? How long until it expires?

Directions: Listen to the information and answer the questions.

1. We are expecting about 100 walkers. They will start and finish at this point. All the volunteers have checked in and have taken a flag and instructions and are going to their posts. The water bottles and T-shirts are being unloaded now.
   What is the event? What are the volunteers carrying?
2. How long has the little light been on? You definitely need oil, and you are lucky that it didn't cause any damage to your engine. Don't ever ignore that light again.
   What light is the speaker referring to? Why shouldn't it be ignored?
3. I don't know that I would recommend it. The soup was really salty and the rolls were cold. The rest of the meal was pretty good, but the waitress was not very attentive. I had to ask for more water and she forgot I asked for the salad dressing on the side.
   What was the speaker talking about? How was the service?
4. The base of the lamp was cracked when I pulled it out of the box. I didn't even try to put it together. I have the receipt and I expect you to either refund my money or replace it with an undamaged one. If you can't do that, I want to see the manager.
   Who is the speaker talking to? What is the problem?
5. Do you think Uncle John is OK? He was really short with me. Then he went off and sat by himself. Do you think he and his son are still having some disagreements about running the shop?
   What kind of a mood is Uncle John in? Who runs the shop?
6. OK, Jody, we won't get there until 3:00, so you should have plenty of time to get back from class. When are you going to pack the rest of your stuff? Sure, we'll bring boxes, but I'm also bringing some putty, a small vacuum, some Simple Green, and a big sponge.
   Why are they going to see Jody? What do you think the putty is for?
7. William Handler is getting my vote. He agrees with me that there is far too much development going on and not enough laws to protect the residents. He recognizes we need to change with the times but to also remember we are mainly a residential, not business, community.
   Why is the speaker voting for Handler? What position could Handler be running for?
8. Your assignment next week will be to read two chapters in the text. There will be a 50-point quiz on Tuesday. In addition, your essays are due next Friday. You should have already picked your celebrity and be researching them in regards to their relationship with the media, paparazzi, and gossip magazines.
   Who would be speaking? What is the subject of the essay and when is it due?
9. You picked a bad time to call and anyhow, I am not interested. I do not make commitments over the phone nor do I give out personal information. I told you no. Three times I said "no." Good-bye.
   What type of call is this? How would you have handled it?
10. There will be no formal briefing today. The president is spending the day in private meetings and then he will join his wife and children at his in-laws for a family birthday dinner. I will now open the session up for questions.
    Who is the speaker? Where will the president be this evening?

11. I was going to drive but gas is so expensive, I decided to look into airfares. If I had made my reservations two days ago, I would have gotten a good deal, but the prices went up. There is no way I can fly now. So I'm back to driving.
    How is the speaker going to travel? Why?

12. Do these feel comfortable? Try walking around in them. They look nice and they have good cushioning. I don't have an 8 in black, but do you want to try an 8½?
    What is the speaker referring to? What color was asked for?

13. No, you cannot have another cookie. You will spoil your dinner. You can't be that hungry since you already had three cookies and a full glass of milk. Why don't you take your brother and go play in the yard?
    Who is probably speaking and to whom? Why won't the person give a cookie?

14. I would like to make a toast to the best sister in the world and my new brother-in-law. I hope your days with Todd are as happy as mine have been with Julie. Todd, you are one lucky man. The best advice I can give you is to always agree with her and keep your sense of humor.
    Where does the conversation take place? What is the advice and what do you think of it?

15. How about those Pistons? They are really something—12 behind in the second period and now they can't miss. If they keep this pace up, they will really roll over the Lakers by at least 12.
    What is being talked about? Who is predicted to win?

16. I do like the layout, but it's bigger than I expected. Although I'd love to have the space, I'm not crazy about having to clean it. And it doesn't have a mudroom or half-bath on the main floor, and I think we really need that.
    What is the speaker referring to? What does the speaker want that is missing?

17. Dr. Downing is a practicing neurosurgeon at Bownett Hospital. She has had numerous research grants and has distinguished herself in the area of minimally invasive surgical options for brain tumors. She heads the Bownett Brain Tumor Center and is vice-president of the Michigan Neurosurgical Association. Please give her a warm welcome.
    What is the speaker doing? What is the doctor's specialty?

18. I'm sorry, but I can't make it for Thanksgiving. I have to work Friday and Saturday, so I would have to pay a lot to fly in and out on Thursday and that wouldn't make sense. But I'll see you in four weeks, and that will go by faster than you think.
    When will the speaker be in town? Why isn't the speaker coming now?

19. So you say that on the night in question you saw Mr. Flynn run out of the building and across the street into a car. It has been established that it was raining that night and the only streetlight was 100 feet away. And you testified that from where you were standing you could not see the man's face. So my question is, how could you possibly know that the person you saw was Mr. Flynn?
    Who is the speaker? Why does the speaker doubt the person could identify Mr. Flynn?

20. But sir, I was just keeping up with traffic. I was in the slow lane and there was a car that was right behind me and I felt like he was pushing me. I was afraid he was going to rear-end me so I had to speed up to keep him off my tail.
    What was the speaker's excuse? Who was the speaker talking to?

Directions: Listen to the information and answer the questions.

1. John left for work at 7:30. He stopped and got a paper. He drove two more miles and picked up Paul, his carpool buddy.
   Who is the passenger? What was his first stop?
2. As part of last year's new landscaping, three rhododendron bushes were planted last summer near the door. Two of the bushes have brown droopy leaves and it doesn't look like they survived the winter. I think we should replace all three with a heartier bush.
   How many survived the winter? What is the plan?
3. The splint is definitely better than a cast. At least I can take it off and shower. And the splint is flexible enough so I can still write with it on. It was a stupid accident. I should never have tried to break the fall with my arm.
   What was probably the result of the fall? What are the benefits of a splint?
4. The Paynes drove to Florida from Ohio last year for the first time with their two kids and a dog. They said they would never do that again. The scenery was nice, but there was so much construction and so many detours that it took them seven hours longer than they had estimated.
   How many were in the car? Why did it take them longer than expected?
5. Because of the recent weather, the weeds have just shot up all over the yard. There are mushrooms growing near the back and dandelions all over the rest of the lawn. Something has to be done about the brown spots that get bigger every year. Maybe we should call a weed-control service.
   Name two things that are a problem in the lawn. What has happened to the brown spots?
6. The Taylors have two weeks off in July this year. They are spending one week at the lake, and the second week they will stay home. They said they have a lot of work they need to do around the house and especially in the yard.
   When is the Taylors' vacation? Where will they spend the first week?
7. I'm so excited the Johnsons are returning from St. Louis. He has been transferred back to headquarters here. She called and wants to know if there are any houses for sale. They would love to come back to the old neighborhood. The company will put him up in a hotel until they find a house, and then she and girls will move out.
   Where do the Johnsons live now? Where do they want to live?
8. There is a huge grand opening for the new mall on Saturday. Part of the parking lot is being turned into a big game area and will have music, contests where you can win big money-off coupons from the stores, hot dogs and hamburgers, and booths with all kinds of free samples.
   What is the reason for the celebration? How can you win coupons?
9. Barb was sick all night, but she feels much better today even though she said she's only going to have liquids. Based on her symptoms, she thinks she probably had food poisoning. Everyone but Barb had meat loaf for dinner. She had leftover chicken salad. She plans on throwing the rest of it out.
   What was the matter with Barb? What does she think caused her problem?
10. I really need a new leather couch. This one is about 20 years old and the springs are shot. The original cream color is now more like light brown. There is a stain on the side, and one of the arms has somehow collapsed. At least it doesn't have any rips.
    What needs to be replaced? What is wrong with the arm?

11. I'm going to have a home jewelry party next Monday night. You might want to work late, make plans with one of your buddies, or at least watch TV in the bedroom. That is, unless you would like to buy me all kinds of jewelry. In that case, you are welcome to join us.
    What and when is the event? What options was the person given?

12. People crowded around Jan to congratulate her on her win. She won the primary and will go up against the incumbent in November. She hopes her stands on local control and lowered property assessments will help her win voters. She hopes she can convince them that her Democratic opponent is fiscally irresponsible.
    What does Jan want if she wins? What do you think she is running for?

13. We've got a foursome to play Oak Hills on Saturday. I'll pick you up at 2:00 so we can be there in time to warm up before our 3:12 teetime. Is it OK if I use your old seven wood? I am thinking of getting one or, if I like it, maybe you'd want to sell it to me.
    What are they going to do Saturday? What is the club that was discussed?

14. Rick went to the hardware store to pick up some primer and a roller pan. While he was there, he ran into Mike, who he hadn't seen for about five years. Mike had gotten a divorce two years ago and is living in an apartment in Troy.
    What was Rick getting at the store? What was new with Mike?

15. I've been on this diet for one month and I've only lost four pounds. I have cut back on carbs and I haven't had any desserts. I walk one mile every day and three times a week I'm doing weight training. I am so discouraged, and that really makes me want to eat more.
    How much weight has the person lost? What exercise has the person been doing?

16. Business has been so good on Saturday that the farmer's market will now open Sunday mornings from 7:00 to 11:00. New vendors with fresh-cut flowers and baked goods will be added on Sunday only. If the organizers hear there is enough interest, they might even add a small flea market.
    What are the new hours of operation? What are the possible plans to expand?

17. On the way home from the movie, Mark and his date stopped at the Dairy Queen. They ordered two Blizzards in a bag so they could take them to Quarton Lake. It was a perfect night to sit on the dock, talk, and eat ice cream.
    What three places did they go? What did they order?

18. Dawn did quite well at the neighborhood yard sale. She sold all of the baby clothes, the crib, and stroller. She was happy to get $100 for both the recliner and dresser. She didn't sell the set of china, but she knew she had priced it high. She got a total of $232 for all the rest of the kitchen items.
    What did Dawn not sell? What did she sell for $100?

19. Wayne was in a hurry to finish his tax returns. He was very frustrated because he couldn't locate some of the receipts for his charitable contributions. He knew he had at least five more. One of the missing letters was from the American Heart Association thanking him for his $500 donation.
    What was Wayne doing? How many receipts is he missing?

20. Tom decided he was going to switch from contacts to glasses. The contacts were irritating his eyes and they were just too much trouble. He is at a stage where most of his friends are wearing glasses so he feels in good company. Other than sunglasses, he has never picked out glasses and is concerned about what will look good on him.
    Why is Tom switching to glasses? What is his main concern?

Directions: Listen to the information and answer the questions.

1. This is Barnes & Noble calling. Your special book order has arrived. The book is *Small Ways to Reduce Big Stress*. You can pick it up at the main desk anytime after 5:00 today.
   Why would someone order this book? When can you pick it up?
2. Raffle tickets are $10 each or six for $50. Don't forget, the grand prize is a new Dell laptop computer valued at $2,400.
   How many tickets do you get for $50? What is the value of the grand prize?
3. Your appointment is Thursday, November 10 at 9:30 with Dr. Hunt. Please bring your script and a copy of your X-rays and give them to the receptionist when you sign in.
   What type of appointment is this? What should you bring with you?
4. The address of Barb's retirement party is 6421 E. Somerset Avenue, apartment C-4. Take the stairs up and turn right.
   How do you get to C-4? What is the occasion?
5. Mary has to cancel your trim at 5:30 on Wednesday. She wants to know if you can reschedule that to Monday at 6:15. Please call and let us know.
   When can Mary see you? What is Mary's job?
6. Cell-tech wants to be your phone company. Call 1-888-463-2000, extension 14 to speak with Rita about saving money on your local and long-distance calls.
   Who is calling? Who do you call and what is her extension?
7. I'll pick you up tomorrow morning bright and early at 6:00. Jenny is going to pack some nuts and granola bars. I'll bring a cooler with water and juice. If we can get off before rush hour, we should be able to make it to Cedar Point by lunch.
   Who is bringing drinks? Where is the group going?
8. Your four Tigers tickets are being held at the box office under the name of Nick. Please bring a check or cash for $62.42. You have unobstructed bleacher seats.
   Do these seats sound like a good deal? How many tickets were ordered?
9. Would you like to come for dinner Friday night? It'll be very informal. We're going to grill some burgers. I'll have leftover appetizers, potatoes, and cake from Ron's birthday the night before. We'll expect you both at 6:30 unless I hear from you. Don't bring a thing unless you want to pick up a movie.
   What is on the menu? What time should you arrive?
10. This is your mother. So is everything all right? Why haven't you called? Your sister said you were gone for the weekend. Where did you go? She also said you were dating a really nice girl. When were you going to tell me?
    Who was the mother calling and why? How did she find out the person was dating?
11. The paint you have chosen is Benjamin Moore. The color is pale khaki in a semi-gloss finish. One gallon will cover about 65 square feet and should be enough for your powder room. One quart of any white flat paint should be fine for the ceiling.
    How much paint will you buy all together? What colors are you buying?

12. I called to let you know we are going to be late. There is a detour on 696. When we realized the road was closed, it was too late to get off and take an alternate route. Once we get past Orchard Road, I think it will open up and we'll make good time. You can expect us to be about a half-hour late. Save us some seats, but go ahead and order. Don't wait—I'm sure you are hungry.
    Where were the people meeting? What was the problem on 696?

13. Thanks so much for offering to take care of things while we are in Florida. We get a morning and an evening paper, so if you could stop by on your way home from work and take the papers inside that would be great. And please water the plants on Wednesday. I left the watering can on the counter and all the plants are in the kitchen.
    When will the papers be brought inside? When should the plants be watered?

14. Commencement will start at 10:00 A.M. in Chrysler Auditorium. Families must be seated by 9:45. Graduation should last approximately two hours. Pictures following the ceremony must be taken outside in the park across the street because the auditorium must be immediately cleared to prepare for the next event.
    Where is the ceremony? Why can't pictures be taken in the auditorium?

15. I am so glad you were able to come to my bridal shower. I know it was a long drive, but it was great having you there. Thanks so much for the toaster. It is the nicest one I've seen. We eat bagels and English muffins a lot so the wide slots will be perfect, and the fact it can toast four pieces at once is a bonus.
    Why were gifts being given? What is special about the toaster?

16. This is Rita from Pottery Barn. The pillows you wanted have come in from our store in Grand Rapids. However, two of the pillows are mint green, and two are Pottery Barn green. You will need to come in with your swatches to see which green you want before we order more.
    Where were the pillows ordered? Why does the shade of green matter?

17. The Purple Heart will be in your neighborhood the week of May 8. Please leave any clothing, shoes, or small toys but not food or eyeglasses in plastic bags on your porch. The truck will take the items and leave you a receipt for tax purposes. Your generosity will help others in need.
    Why would you put items on your porch? What are two things they will not take?

18. The Board of Directors meets quarterly in February, June, September, and November. The meeting is always the third Monday of the month from 2:00 until the agenda is completed. There will be a dinner break if needed.
    When does the board meet? How long do you think the meetings last?

19. This is to let you know that your fax did not go through. I am calling the number on the cover sheet, and it was the only sheet that came through. That sheet indicated there were five pages. Please refax to Kelly in Purchasing.
    What was wrong with the faxed information? How did the people who originally faxed learn there was a problem?

20. I am calling from Dr. Napp's office. We just called in your prescription for an antibiotic cream. It should be ready for you in an hour. It is important to use this exactly as directed. Call us if your skin becomes very itchy or red because it could be an allergic reaction.
    Where would a doctor's office call in a prescription for you? When should the person using the cream be concerned?

Directions: Listen to the information and answer the questions.

1. An easy way to clean a blender is to fill it about halfway with water. Add a few drops of liquid dish soap. Cover the blender and turn it on medium for about a minute. Rinse it and dry.
   What is the problem to be solved? What do you add to the water? Do you run the blender on low, medium, or high?

2. To remove a broken lightbulb from a socket, gently push a bar of soap into the remaining jagged pieces. Then you can use the soap as a kind of handle to gently guide the bulb out of the socket.
   What is the problem to be solved? Do you break off pieces of the lightbulb? Do you twist or gently pull the bulb straight out?

3. You can use kitty litter to get rid of oil spots on a garage floor. Pour some kitty litter over the oil spot. The important part is to smash the litter into the oil with your foot. Leave it until the next day, then sweep up the mess. This may need to be done a few times before the litter will absorb all of the oil.
   What is the problem to be solved? Should you mix the kitty litter with water? How long do you leave the kitty litter on before removing it?

4. There is a painless way to help the pain with an ingrown toenail. Take toenail clippers and cut a small V shape into the middle of the nail on the ingrown toe. The idea is that the nail will grow inward toward the V you cut rather than at the ends where the nail grows into your flesh.
   What is the problem to be solved? Where do you cut a V? After the slash, how is your nail supposed to grow?

5. If your hands get cold outside in the winter, try this idea. Buy a pair of rubber or latex examination gloves at a drugstore. Wear the gloves under your regular gloves and your hands should be much warmer. It works on the same principle as wet suits that keep divers warm.
   What is the problem to be solved? What product should you buy? How and when do you wear them?

6. There is an easy way to make squeaky wooden floors quiet. Find a board that squeaks. Sprinkle some talcum powder or baby powder along the cracks between the boards and rub it in until the cracks are filled. Either the noise will be gone, or it will be much quieter than before.
   What is the problem to be solved? What product do you need to have on hand? Do you use the powder on the squeaking board or between two boards?

7. After a few uses, glass vases can look cloudy and gray. To make the glass look clear again, fill it with water. Plop in two Alka-Seltzer tablets and let them dissolve. Watch for the fizzing. After all the fizzing has stopped, rinse out the vase a few times with plain water. Let it air dry or use a soft towel and the vase should be sparkly and clear.
   What is the problem to be solved? What do you put in the vase? Do you stir the mixture or let it sit?

8. If your photographs are sticking together, there is a way to get them apart without damaging them. Put the photos in the freezer for 10 to 20 minutes. Bring them out and try to gently pry them apart with a butter knife or a similar blunt instrument. If the photographs won't come apart, put them back in the freezer and try again after a few minutes.
   What is the problem to be solved? If you don't have a butter knife handy, what could you use instead? Do you put the photos in the refrigerator or the freezer?

9. Some jewelry pieces can leave a dark mark on your skin or your clothing. The jewelry backs leave the marks as they rub against fabric or skin all day. To avoid this problem, paint the back of the piece of jewelry with clear nail polish. Let it dry before wearing it again and the problem will be solved. The nail polish will need to be reapplied every so often as it will wear off with time.
   What is the problem to be solved? What product do you need for this solution? What part of the jewelry do you paint?

10. If you are making a recipe and you don't have an egg, you can substitute either of the following for one egg: one teaspoon cornstarch mixed with three tablespoons extra liquid, or use two tablespoons oil plus one tablespoon water.
   What is the problem to be solved? What do you mix with cornstarch? What do you add to one tablespoon water?

11. If you have a barbecue grill or oven rack with grease and burned-on food, there is an easy way to clean it. Place the cool rack on your lawn overnight. The dew along with the enzymes in the grass will help loosen the burned-on food and grease. It should be much easier to clean with hot, soapy water the next day.
   What is the problem to be solved? Where do you put the rack? Do enzymes in the air or the grass help the cleaning process?

12. There is an easier and cheaper way to hold up plants than to tie them using twist-ties. Get an old plastic bag. The size is not important, and it doesn't matter if it was used before. Use scissors to cut the bag into strips about one inch wide. Use the strips to tie the stem of the plant and a stick together so the plant will grow upright.
   What is the problem to be solved? Can you use a plastic grocery bag? Should the strips be one inch long or one inch wide?

13. Here are some different food ideas: (1) Use Lifesavers candy around the bottom of the candles on a birthday cake to stop the dripping and to look colorful. (2) Stuff a miniature marshmallow in the bottom of an ice cream cone so it doesn't drip. (3) Freeze leftover wine in ice cube trays so you can add some wine to sauces when you need it. You could also put a few cubes in a tall glass and fill it with club soda for a refreshing spritzer.
   What will using the marshmallow prevent? What is another use for the wine cubes? How could you use Lifesavers on a cake?

14. Your dishwasher should get special treatment at least twice a year. Preheat the water for your dishwasher by running the faucet until it is hot. Dump a pint jar of Tang powdered drink into the bottom of the empty dishwasher. Turn on the dishwasher and run it through an entire cycle. This procedure will remove the build-up of detergent and mineral deposits in the machine.
   What is the problem to be solved? What product do you need and how much of it? How often should you do this process?

15. Experimentation has shown that there are better things than cheese to go in mousetraps. One food mice like is chocolate after-dinner mints. Peanut butter and raw bacon are also recommended. Some people have had success with sticky stale jellybeans.
   What is the problem to be solved? What are three foods to try in a mousetrap? Would you use raw or cooked bacon?

16. There are many ideas for relaxing your body. One of the more unusual ones involves your toes. Lie on your back and wiggle the toes of both feet up and down 12 times. This should relax your entire body. According to reflexology, your toes are a control for your body. So by wiggling them, you are helping to bring a relaxing, free-flowing energy throughout your body.
    What is the problem to be solved? What do you do and for how long? Why does this work?

17. Paul Harvey has talked several times about his "natural" cure for arthritis on his radio show. To make the cure, take a box of golden raisins and place the raisins in a shallow container. You must use white or golden raisins, not dark ones. Totally cover the raisins with gin and put a loose lid on the container. Let the mixture soak a few weeks until the gin has evaporated. Paul says to eat nine of the raisins each day and you will feel better.
    What is the problem to be solved? How much gin do you use? Do you use white, golden, or dark raisins?

18. Do you get irritated with all the insects that are caked on the bumper of your car after a long trip? A way to prevent this from happening is to buy a nonstick cooking spray such as Pam and completely spray the front of your car. This will keep the bugs from sticking when they hit it at a high rate of speed. You can easily remove the spray with a good car washing.
    What is the problem to be solved? What do you put on the front of your car? Do you remove the spray by wiping it off or washing it off?

19. The following is an unusual cure for a sore throat. Finely chop an onion and put it into a container with a lid that seals. Sprinkle two to four tablespoons of sugar over the onions. Seal the lid and place the container in a cool place until a juice forms. Drain off a tablespoon or two of juice and swallow it every four hours until the sore throat is gone.
    What is the problem to be solved? What ingredients do you need? How often do you use the concoction?

20. How do you know if a new dish is safe to put in a microwave oven? Here is a solution. Fill the dish half full of water and set it next to your microwave oven. Turn the oven on high and let it run for one minute. Next, feel your dish. If the dish is hot, do not use it in the microwave. If the dish is warm, it can be used for reheating at 80 percent power. If the dish stays at room temperature, you know it is totally safe for the microwave.
    What is the problem to be solved? What does it mean if the dish is hot? When the microwave is running, should the dish be inside or next to the oven?

Directions: Listen to the story. There is something that does not make sense or is just not quite right in the story. Point out what does not belong.

1. It was a hot, humid day. The air conditioner was working full-time to keep the house somewhat cool. The only way to survive a hot shower was to take a quick one. Some relief from the heat came from closing the blinds to keep the sun out and opening the windows to bring in a breeze.

2. Five friends from Carol's office planned a baby shower for her. They wanted to give her some practical gifts since this is her first baby. They each chipped in money to buy one large gift. Carol was so surprised when they presented her with a beach umbrella and picnic basket full of munchies and snacks.

3. It is not well known that Abraham Lincoln was working on a draft of the Gettysburg Address and solicited the help of Thomas Jefferson. Lincoln and Jefferson collaborated on the paragraph about emancipation.

4. Mary was asked to be a bridesmaid in her brother's wedding. Mary will be carrying his ring on a pillow as she walks down the aisle. His best man will walk with the other bridesmaids.

5. A revolutionary new diet has hit the markets. After years of testing and analysis, the FDA has approved Alloff, a pill by Pfizer, as an alternative to dieting. This pill's power lies in its ability to dissolve fat cells. Now no one will ever have an excuse to be overweight again.

6. Fort Lauderdale has a national reputation as a great place to enjoy the sun and nightlife. The population explodes in the spring as northerners flock to Lauderdale beaches during their Thanksgiving break. It is especially popular for college students doing research papers.

7. It is important for John to catch the 8:05 evening flight from Detroit to Memphis. That flight should arrive in Memphis at 9:40. He can rent a cab at the airport and drive directly to Mobile Tech Industries in time for a late afternoon meeting.

8. The Kings have a summer home on Lake Michigan. It is about 50 feet from the water and has a rocky shoreline. It is a natural lake and no power boats are allowed. We find it peaceful and quiet except for the first week in July when the annual hydroplane races take place.

9. The second Tuesday of every month, the "ladies of Newgate" get together for Bunco. They all live on Newgate Street and all work late on Tuesday evenings. One person hosts the party and three people bring appetizers. Everyone brings drinks. They get together at six and talk and play for a few hours. Since there are twelve of them, each hosts one month out of the year.

10. Meijer is having a clearance sale on patio furniture. Umbrella tables usually at $230 are going for $185. Web mesh chairs are on sale at $75 each or you can get a set of four for $380. Hammocks with collapsible stands are $210, on sale from $300. Come early for the best selection.

11. The Chocolate Ball will honor those who have given their time and money during the past year to the local chapter of the Diabetes Association. This year's ball will take place at the Hyatt and feature an all-chocolate buffet. All foods, including appetizers, salads, and entreés, will have some form of chocolate as an ingredient. As in the past, 100 honored diabetics will be given tickets to the event.

12. If you are like most people, your closets are bursting at the seams. Closet Control is waiting for your call. Our control freaks will come and evaluate your situation. They will recommend a system of shelves, drawers, rods, and baskets to give you the most flexibility and space that your dimensions allow. A written plan will be provided, and, upon your prepayment, we will immediately empty your closet and have our system completely installed within two hours of your signature. Call us for an appointment.

13. Although it is too early to know for sure, it appears that the fire broke out in the garage. Firefighters responded after getting a call at 10:03 from within the home. Because of the winds, a second unit was called in as backup to help at 10:35. The blaze was contained by noon, however, one truck remained as a precaution. Luckily no one was home at the time and there were no injuries.

14. Rising gas costs are thought to be a direct result of the slumping sales in the high-fuel consumption sport utility vehicles. The car industry has responded by experimenting with alternative fuels and improving mileage in all vehicles. Statistics have shown that Americans have responded by driving less and for shorter periods of time on the road, and by increasing their travel by air.

15. Miller's 21st birthday was a milestone. A few years ago, no one would have thought he would have made it to this day. Miller has attention deficit disorder, a life-threatening disease that was diagnosed at birth. Doctors gave Miller a 50/50 chance of graduating from high school. Miller has lots to celebrate because he is not only alive but will be graduating magna cum laude from Stanford in June. He is an example of a modern medical miracle.

16. We really need this rain. It has been dry for almost a month. The grass is brown, flowers are blooming in black and white rather than colors, and there is dust all over. The forecast shows a wide band of showers and thunderstorms heading this way. For once, I hope we get drenched.

17. This picture is of my great-grandfather. This is the original photograph and wood frame. He was born sometime in the early 1800s and died in 1951. He and my great grandmother lived in Minneapolis where he worked as a bookkeeper. They had seven children of which my grandfather was the youngest boy.

18. I just finished reading *Good-bye Gucci*. It just came out and I got one of the first copies. I loved it! The book was based on a true story and written by a member of a family that moved from a penthouse in New York City to a working dairy farm in upstate New York. It's been on the *New York Times* bestseller list for three months. I'm sure you can find it wherever books are sold.

19. Joe asked if I would call you and let you know he won't be leaving work until 11:00 tonight. He is working another half-shift and couldn't leave the register to call you. He also said that if you needed anything at the mall to let him know. He's planning on stopping there to look at shoes on his way home.

20. Did you hear about the lady who lives in the blue house that sits way back from the road? I heard she was arrested yesterday after police raided her home. They received a tip from someone that she was feeding stray cats and finding them new homes. Based on the evidence, they expect she will get at least a citation and maybe jail time for saving the lives of those cats.

Directions: Listen to the information and answer the questions.

1. The mail was mostly ads, but it had a few surprises. An unexpected dividend check came from a stock split as well as an invitation to a surprise 50th birthday party. The rest of the mail was bills, a *Consumers Report* magazine, and a new VISA card.
   Why was there a check in the mail? What invitation was in the mail? Name all the things that came in the mail.

2. When Anne returned home from shopping, she drove her car into the garage and went in through that door. She put her packages and purse down in the kitchen and walked to the bathroom. On the way she checked to see if the ficus needed watering.
   Where had Anne been? What did she do with her purse? What did she do last?

3. The reporter kept breaking up during the shooting of the piece. The horse behind him kept nuzzling around his ear and it tickled. It looked like the seventh take would be good, but during her final sentence, the horse pushed the reporter's head forward and threw her off-balance. One more take.
   What was causing so many retakes? Why did the reporter keep laughing? What could have been done to prevent the problem?

4. Alex had his first Little League game on Saturday morning. He was at bat three times and made two hits and struck out once. He started playing infield but the coach switched him to first base after five innings. He made some great outs, and he should feel very good about how he did.
   When was Alex told to switch positions? How many hits did he make? What game was he playing?

5. There is a family of skunks that have taken up residence in the yard. The poor dog has now been "skunked" twice in the last four days. It is time to bring in the professionals with some humane traps. This furry family needs to be relocated to a place where they will be more appreciated.
   How many times has the dog been skunked? What will be done about the problem? What will happen to the skunks that are caught?

6. Tom Clark opened the Whistle Stop restaurant in 2002. Since then, it has gained a loyal following of patrons who love the home-cooked meals. Clark is known for his pies overflowing with fresh fruit and especially his melt-in-your-mouth dark chocolate cream pie with real whipped cream.
   Who owns the restaurant? What type of food is it known for? Describe the chocolate pie.

7. Aunt Ellen really amazed me when I heard her play the piano. I had no idea she was so good. I knew she could sing because she is in the Symphony Choir and their auditions are hard. I actually got tears in my eyes when she was playing and singing *Amazing Grace*.
   What are her musical talents? What did she sing? Why was the speaker surprised?

8. I'm really worried about Erik. All he does is work. Most days he doesn't get home until 11:00 at night and then he's gone again at 7:00 in the morning. He has no social life, and if it weren't for some tennis at the club, he wouldn't leave his office. He says he's fine and that he needs to do the job. There is something very wrong with his reasoning; no job is more important than someone's life and health.
   What are his usual work hours? What kind of exercise does he get? What would you say to Erik if you had the opportunity?

9. Jane took home nine samples of upholstery material for the chairs. She is having a hard time figuring out what kind of pattern she wants. Her top choices are the paisley print and the solid, textured suede. She was able to eliminate five of the choices pretty easily. The other two are striped and she is afraid they might show dirt too easily.
   What are her top two choices? Why didn't she like the stripes? Why is she looking at fabrics?

10. I want to send flowers to my wife for her birthday. She really likes tulips but they are not in season. She can't stand red or orange flowers. A variety of any other colors would be great. Please slip in one pink carnation—it's a little joke between us. And one more thing—she really likes purple.
    What is the occasion for the flowers? What color does she not like? What flowers and colors could you put in the bouquet?

11. Hannah went next door to see if she could borrow some milk to make biscuits. No one was home on either side, so she gave up. She figured if she had to go to the store she might as well shop for the next few days, so she sat down and made a list.
    What was she going to make? What ingredient did she need? What could Hannah do instead of going to the store?

12. It looks pretty chilly and dreary now, but it is supposed to clear up by noon. The high later this afternoon is going to be 72 degrees and the forecast is for a 75 percent chance of the sun coming out. It sounds like a great time to wash the car.
    What is the weather like now? What is the chance the sun will come out? What is the forecasted high?

13. The factory will shut down for good on Friday at 4:00 P.M. About 100 people took the early retirement offer and about another 50 were given jobs in the Warren plant. While it is a sad occasion, all 400 employees knew it was coming for at least a year.
    When will the factory close? How many people will transfer to another plant? What would you suspect other plant workers did before the closing?

14. Tom has a deep gash in his arm. He was holding a bottle of pop when he fell. It smashed and a big piece of glass cut his arm. I wrapped the arm in a towel and told him to keep it above his head. That worked a little but it was still bleeding so I thought we'd better go to Emergency to have it checked. Three hours later we arrived home with 22 stitches in Tom's arm as a reminder of the event.
    How did Tom injure himself? Why was it decided to go to the hospital? What happened at the hospital?

15. Dan Winter is a sales rep for Turner Paint Supplies. His territory is the state of Indiana. He puts more than 35,000 miles a year on his vehicle. He travels from place to place with his samples loaded in the van. It sounds lonely, but it must pay off for him because he is almost the top salesperson in the country.
    What is the name of the company? How many miles does he put on his vehicle? Where is his territory?

16. Last year the Hendersons went skiing in Vermont. They rented a small condo that slept eight. It had a great view of the slopes and the backdoor opened right onto the base of the hill. Although the condo had a microwave and a small refrigerator, they had their dinners in the lodge sitting in front of the huge two-story stone fireplace.
    Where did they go on vacation? Why did they eat dinner in the lodge? Describe what you know about the condo.

17. The Bloomfield Club has several requirements for membership. You must have a letter of recommendation from at least two people who have been members in good standing for at least 10 years. You must have proof that you have volunteered a minimum of 15 hours a month in the community for a recognized and worthy cause. You must reside in the city of Bloomfield and be at least 25 years old.
    How many requirements does the club have for membership? How long does someone have to be a member before nominating a potential member? What is the volunteer requirement?

18. The publishing firm of Reed and Wright has published a popular series of books on furniture. The first book, published last year, focuses on the history of furniture making in the United States. Two more books are due out by the end of the year. The series editors have brought together experts in both antique and contemporary furniture.
    Who would be interested in this series? By the end of this year, how many of the books should be available? What is the focus of the series?

19. Workers just finished a number of new improvements at Pembroke Park. The old splintery wood benches were replaced with new dark green metal ones. There are now four picnic tables with seating near the benches. The new play structures are great. They are colorful and full of things to walk through, hang on, and slide down. The walking trail has been widened and has a thick new layer of wood chips.
    Describe the play structures. What were the benches replaced with? What happened to the trail?

20. As Pam walked down the hall to her office, she noticed a woman watching her. She turned and smiled at the woman who then said, "Aren't you Linda's daughter?" Surprised, she said, "Yes, how did you know that?" The woman said, "I'm Mrs. Daly. I used to babysit for you when you lived on Harris Street."
    Why did Pam smile at the woman? How did the woman know Pam? What was Pam's mother's name?

Directions: Listen to the information and answer the questions.

1. Baby Wipes have a number of uses. 1) They are great for shining faucets and dashboards in cars. 2) They can clean and polish leather shoes. 3) They can also be used to blot up stains that are still wet. 4) They are a good cloth to use to dust off wood surfaces.
   What product is this about? What was the second use? How are they used on stains?

2. Bounce Fabric Softener has a number of different uses. 1) The sheets can be used as mosquito repellant. Tie a sheet of Bounce through a belt loop or a buttonhole. 2) Bounce can deodorize your shoes. Place a sheet in each shoe and leave it overnight. The shoes should smell much better in the morning. 3) Rub a sheet of Bounce over a dog's or cat's fur to pick up loose hairs.
   Besides the idea listed, how else could you wear Bounce as a mosquito repellant? How would you use Bounce to make your shoes smell better?

3. Here are some tips about raw eggs: 1) A stale egg will sink if it is put into a pot of water while a fresh one will float. 2) If you add vinegar to the water when you are making hard-boiled eggs, it will help seal the egg so the shell won't crack. 3) If you don't know if an egg is raw or hard-boiled, spin it. If it spins easily, it is hard boiled, but if it wobbles around, it is raw.
   How can you tell if an egg is stale? How can you tell if an egg is hard-boiled? What does vinegar have to do with hard-boiled eggs?

4. Pumpkins have other uses than just for jack-o'-lanterns. 1) A few spoonfuls of canned pumpkin will help puppies that have diarrhea. 2) Three ounces of pumpkin seeds crushed and mixed into a paste with honey and eaten daily is said to help prostate disorders. 3) As a remedy for very dry skin or eczema, mix pumpkin puree, nutmeg, and almond oil. Apply to the skin and rinse off after about 15 minutes.
   What is the second idea? What do you apply to very dry skin? What do you give to puppies with diarrhea?

5. Several remedies to clean areas on a painted wall are: 1) Use an art gum eraser on the spots. 2) Use some baking soda on a damp rag and rub the spot gently. 3) Use non-gel toothpaste on a cloth or the tip of your finger. 4) Try hair spray or rubbing alcohol to remove ink or Magic Marker.
   What supplies would you need to try all the methods? What will the remedies supposedly do? What would you use if a child drew on a wall with a felt-tip pen?

6. Most people know how to use tweezers to pull out splinters. Here are some other ideas that should also work: 1) Put tape over the splinter and pull it off. 2) Soak the area in oil before removing the splinter. 3) Put a bit of Elmer's glue on the splinter and let it dry, then peel off the dried glue. 4) Put a small piece of uncooked bacon on the splinter. Cover it with a bandage and leave it overnight. By the next morning, the salt and grease should have brought the splinter to the surface.
   What were the remedies for the previous question? Why is a bandage used? How and why do you use Elmer's glue?

7. These morning-after hangover remedies are tried and true—at least for some people. 1) Drink a glass of chocolate milk along with a vitamin and three aspirin. 2) Drink a Coke with a piece of cold pizza. 3) Eat a peanut butter, honey, and banana sandwich on white bread. 4) Mix equal quantities of room-temperature V-8 juice and club soda and drink it slowly.
   What is taken with a vitamin? What are you supposed to drink at room temperature? What kind of sandwich is supposed to be a cure?

8. Changes in air pressure in a plane can cause your ears to pop, plug up, or hurt. Some of the more popular remedies to help this include: 1) Constantly chew gum. 2) Take a decongestant half an hour before the plane takes off. 3) Wear earplugs during the flight. 4) If your ears are plugged, pinch your nostrils and gently blow out your nose.
   What three effects can a change in air pressure have on your ears? What things can you do that do not involve medicine? What is a brand-name medication you could take and when would you take it?

9. Here are some ways to chop an onion without crying: 1) Cut the onion under running water. 2) Heat the onion in a microwave for one minute before cutting it. 3) Hold a piece of bread in your mouth while chopping the onion. 4) Chop the onion inside a plastic bag. 5) Chill the onion for at least an hour in the refrigerator before chopping it.
   How many ideas were listed? What idea uses bread? Which one sounds the best?

10. Some of the more unusual uses for Coca-Cola are: 1) Pour Coke over a jellyfish bite to relieve the sting. 2) Pour Coke over your skin to help you get a tan. 3) Pour Coke over car battery terminals to get rid of corrosion. 4) Add Coke to a load of wash along with the detergent, to remove grease stains. 5) Soak a cloth in Coke and press it on a rusted bolt for a few minutes to loosen it.
    Which ideas would you try? Why would you add Coke to a washing machine? How are the third and the last ideas similar?

11. There are five ways to clean copper pots. The first one uses a spray bottle that has a mixture of vinegar and 3 tablespoons of salt in it. Spray the mixture on the pot and let it stand a few minutes, then rub it clean. You can also use toothpaste, Worcestershire sauce, or ketchup. Put one of these on a paper towel or rag and rub it over the copper. The final idea is to dip half a lemon in salt and rub it over the surface of the pot.
    Name five ingredients that were mentioned. What do you put in a spray bottle? What was the final idea?

12. If you have mosquito bites, here are some ways you can take the itch out of them: 1) Slap the bite instead of itching it. 2) Dab the bite with vinegar as soon as you can after you have been bitten. 3) Rub the bite with non-gel mint toothpaste. 4) Apply rubbing alcohol or lavender oil to the bite. 5) Make a paste of meat tenderizer and water, and apply it to the bite.
    What will the remedies help? Which one does not require equipment? What is the fourth idea?

13. If you are out of kitty litter and need a substitute, try using shredded newspaper sprinkled with baking soda. If you are out of brass polish, use ketchup. If you are out of chrome cleaner, use vinegar. If you don't have any eyeglass cleaner but you have vodka, use that instead. If you are out of hair conditioner, try using mayonnaise instead.
    If you were polishing brass and chrome candlesticks, what products from your kitchen could you use? What is a cheap substitute for kitty litter? What was the last idea?

14. There are many ways to cure hiccups besides scaring someone. Other methods that have worked at least once are: 1) Find your Adam's apple and move back to the indented area just above the bones. Apply ice cubes to both sides of this spot. 2) Rub your earlobes. 3) Put your hands and elbows over your head and hold your breath for a count of 20. 4) Pinch your nose shut while you drink a glass of water. 5) Gargle with a mouthful of Coca-Cola.
    How many cures were listed? Which one will you try first? Explain the most complicated one.

15. Garlic lovers can use one of these remedies to get rid of or reduce garlic breath: 1) Eat fresh parsley during the meal in which you are also eating garlic. 2) Make sure everyone you are around has also eaten garlic. 3) Chew on a coffee bean. 4) Suck on a lemon wedge that has been sprinkled with salt. 5) Drink red wine or have a bowl of lime sherbet after the garlic. 6) Brush your teeth, then use a mouthwash.
    What foods are mentioned in the remedies? What are the two things you could chew? What do you do with the lemon?

16. Here are some unusual home remedies for baldness: 1) Scrub the bald area with onions until it becomes red, then apply honey over the redness. Leave it on until the redness disappears. 2) Massage coconut milk into the scalp and roots. Leave it on for a half-hour, then rinse it off with warm water. 3) Wash the hair with cold water and vigorously rub the scalp with your fingertips until it starts to tingle and you feel heat. 4) Grind up lime seeds and peppercorns in equal amounts and make a paste with a small amount of water. Apply that to the bald patches regularly.
    What do you do with coconut milk? What ingredients do you grind up? Which remedy sounds the least likely to work and why?

17. How can you remove a ring that is stuck on your finger? Try these ideas: 1) If your finger is swollen, rub ice over your finger and wait until the swelling goes down before trying anything. 2) Apply lotion, butter, dishwashing liquid, or mayonnaise. 3) Take a long piece of dental floss and slide it under the ring. Begin to wind the floss up your finger and move the ring up as you are winding. 4) Spray Windex or a glass cleaner over the area before trying to slide the ring off. This also cleans the ring.
    Which one should you do first? What are four things you can apply to the finger to help make it easier to slide the ring off? Show how you would use dental floss to get off a ring.

18. There are several things that people should do when storing silver items. 1) Do not wrap silver in newspaper because the ink will remove silver plating. 2) Do not put rubber bands around silver even if it is through layers of paper because the silver will stain. 3) Do not put silver in felt unless the material has been treated and sold as tarnish-preventative felt. 4) Do not store silver in plastic unless it is made of mylar or polyethylene. Other types of plastic will cause pits to form on the surface of the silver.
    Why shouldn't you store silver in newspaper? What types of plastic are fine for storing silver? What are two other items that should not be used for storing silver?

19. Here are four ways to prevent dogs from digging in a yard: 1) Bury some moth ice crystals where the dog usually digs. Dogs do not like their smell. 2) Sprinkle cayenne pepper or hot sauce over the areas where the dog digs. The taste and smell might deter the dog, though some dogs like it. 3) Partially blow up some balloons and bury them around the yard. Cover them lightly with new dirt. This will associate digging there with an unpleasant pop. 4) Fill an empty soft drink can with pebbles and tape off the opening. Stand nearby and watch the dog, but don't interact with it. When the dog begins to dig, throw the can NEAR the dog. You do not want to hit the dog, but you do want to startle it with the noise so that the dog will associate an unpleasant noise with digging.

    How would you use hot sauce or cayenne paper? What could be a problem with using balloons? Why do you need to be careful using the soft drink can?

20. If you have any old tennis balls around the house, there are a number of things you can do with them. 1) They make a great little safe for jewelry. Cut a slit along one of the seams. Squeeze the slit open and place your small valuables inside. Put it in an inconspicuous place or with other sports equipment—just don't let someone use it for games. 2) Add a bunch of tennis balls to your dryer when you are drying a down jacket, pillow, or comforter. The balls will help fluff up the down. 3) With your car parked in your garage, hang a string from the ceiling with a tennis ball on the end that just touches your windshield. This will give you a visual reminder of where to stop the car. 4) If you have a deck, slit four tennis balls and fit them over the feet of your lawn chairs. The balls will keep the legs of the chair from slipping through the openings on the deck.

    If you used a tennis ball as a safe, where would you hide it? What does a tennis ball have to do with a down comforter? What was the last idea and can you think of where else you might use that idea?

Directions: Listen to the information and answer the questions.

1. I will meet you at Bud's Beefsteak Tavern after work on Friday. The Tavern used to be Chang's Chinese and is in the Woodland Square Strip Mall. The mall is on the west side of Woodward near Lincoln in Hunter Heights.
   What kind of food did the restaurant used to serve and what does it serve now? What is the name of the mall where it is located? What city is it in?

2. Please stop at Hillside's on your way home. We need a roll of paper towels, Grey Poupon mustard, a loaf of whole-grain wheat bread, a half-gallon of 1 percent milk, and a big jar of honey-roasted peanuts. Oh, I almost forgot, please get some Tide with the blue cap.
   What type of store is Hillside's? How many items are on the list? What kind of bread should you get?

3. The main responsibilities of the job include scheduling patients for three doctors, getting insurance pre-authorizations, restocking exam rooms, and putting together a weekly calendar. If you are experienced with foot massage, that is a big plus.
   What type of job does this describe? What is a weekly responsibility? What extra skill is desirable?

4. I am letting you know that your home equity loan application for $30,000 is incomplete. We still need a copy of your W-2 forms from last year, and we need the middle name of your mother's father as a password. We also need you to read and initial page 5 at the top and line 13 on page 18. When we have the completed application, we will be able to process the request and have an answer for you in 48 hours.
   What is the person applying for? What password name is needed? Where do you initial?

5. This message will confirm your USAirways ticket from Atlanta to Chicago, Flight 654. The plane is scheduled to leave Atlanta on Thursday, March 3, at 11:00 in the morning. The flight is nonstop arriving at Chicago's Midway Terminal at 2:48 Chicago time. You do not have a seat assignment. Please arrive at the airport at least two hours before flight time.
   Where does the flight originate and land? What time should you be at the airport? What is the date of the flight?

6. This is a reminder from the Quarton Lake Neighborhood Association that our annual Arbor Day walk is this weekend. You must preregister and pay $5 for each walker. We also need to know a T-shirt size for all walkers. Mills Market is donating the T-shirts for the walkers. All proceeds from the event will go to our "Save the Elms" program.
   What is the event? What information is needed and why? What will the money help?

7. The Radisson Plaza Hotel has reserved one room with a king-size bed in your name. The room is on the sixth floor and has an ocean view with a balcony. Per your request, the room will be nonsmoking. You will need to secure the room now with a credit card. If you do not cancel 48 hours in advance, the room rate, taxes, plus a 10 percent cancellation fee will be charged to the card.
   Would this room be acceptable to you if you were traveling? What is the name of the hotel? If you don't cancel and don't arrive, what will happen?

8. Your check #4362 to VISA Bankcard was returned to us for lack of sufficient funds. We will be rebilling for the $215.50 plus a $25 processing fee, a $15 late fee, and any financial charges that have accrued since November 23. Thank you for your business.
   What was the check number? How much more is being charged over the amount of the original bill? When do the finance charges start accruing?

9. This is Dr. Harrison calling to give you the results of Rover's testing. He does not have heartworm or Parvo and his bloodwork came back normal. He does have some parasites, but they can be easily treated with pills. We'll have some ready for you when you stop by. Just crush one pill in his food for the next seven days and he should be fine.
   What type of doctor is calling? What does Rover not have? How should his problem be treated?

10. Pick up the dry cleaning at Star Cleaners. Drop off the movies at King Video Rental. Take the boots to Sam's Shoes and tell them to put new one-inch heels on them. And don't forget to pick up Sarah at school no later than 3:45.
    How many errands were listed? What is Sam supposed to do? When should Sarah be picked up?

11. The estimate of all repairs for your car is $967 including labor. That breaks down to $320 to bump out the dents, $280 to fix the passenger-side exterior mirror, $330 to do touch-up paint work, and $37 to change the oil and check the fluids. You can pick it up after 4:00 today. Call the Service Department if you have questions.
    What is being done to the car? Which work is the most expensive? When will the car be ready?

12. Ken thinks he and his wife are going to dinner Saturday with the Bakers at the Country Grill, but his wife knows differently. Ten other friends will be waiting for him in the Grill's Pheasant Room at 6:45. Ken will arrive at 7:00 and drinks and dinner will follow. Everyone was told not to bring gifts but to bring a poem, photo, card, or good story about Ken.
    What type of event is planned? Specifically where will the event take place? What should each person bring?

13. We have your name on the waiting list for golf lessons. We now have availability in two evening classes. There is an opening in the Short Irons class on Mondays at 7:30 and the Putting Class on Thursdays at 6:00. Both classes have a maximum of six people, last for four weeks, and cost $85. Call if you are interested and ask for Ted. If we do not hear from you in 24 hours, we will call the next person on the list.
    What classes have openings? How long do the classes last? What happens if you do not call back?

14. What would you like to bring to the potluck? I know you don't cook so if you don't want to bring food, we still need drinks, paper cups, and napkins. The main dishes are fried chicken and roll-up sandwiches. If you pick something up, don't get a dessert because we have plenty. We could use some more side dishes or salads—but not tossed salad. What do you feel like doing?
    What type of event is talked about? What items are still needed? What items are not needed?

15. I really appreciate you feeding the cat in the morning. I put the cans and opener out on the counter. You will also see the dry food with a scoop in the bag. Just open the can and empty the whole thing into the dish. Then mix it with one scoop of the dry food. Before you leave, fill up two water bowls with fresh water.
    What food does the cat get? When does the cat get fed? What should you do before leaving?

16. The reason why your phone bill did not show a credit is because the new information did not reach our computer until after the bill was processed. You can expect last month's $35 credit to appear on your next bill. By then, everything will have caught up, and the new special price of $14.95 for Internet services will be listed every month. This special lasts for 12 months.
    How much credit do you get? How long will the deal last? What type of bill is it?

17. We have checked your lawn and noticed a lot of clover, weeds, and bare spots. We recommend our premium lawn care package. That includes six treatments between now and the winter. We also expect you will need special spot treatments for the weeds. We have a deal that if you prepay for the season you will get 15 percent off.
    Who would be leaving this message? How can you get a discount? What does the recommended package include?

18. Guess what! I'm engaged, and wait until you hear how he asked me. We were sitting on his porch and he asked me if I wanted some iced tea. I said OK, and he left. He brought the iced tea back in a tall glass with ice cubes like usual, except it was on a saucer and had a tall spoon in it. I kidded him that it was like being in a fine restaurant and said I was impressed with his presentation. Well, to make a long story short, he had frozen the ring inside one of the ice cubes. I didn't even notice anything until I was almost done and at first, I couldn't tell if it was a bug or worse in the ice cube.
    Was his idea a good one? What did he do to prepare? What did he serve her?

19. Each year, millions suffer needlessly from the pain associated with arthritis. A new over-the-counter pain reliever has been shown to be more effective than any other non-prescription drug in helping people with arthritis live a pain-free life. Ask your local druggist for information on R-Relief—the great new drug for arthritis that comes in pill or capsule form in the bright red bottle.
    What is the name of the drug? Why is it supposedly different? How can you find it on the shelf?

20. I'm returning your call about the bedroom items I have for sale. There is a bedroom set with a dresser, queen-size bed frame and headboard, and two end tables. The wood is dark cherry with polished brass knobs. I would say it has a traditional look. The dresser has two small drawers at the top, then four long ones. The top drawers are velvet lined and not very deep. The bed frame holds the mattress, and the headboard has a curved top with some carvings in it. The end tables each have one drawer with a shelf under it. Everything is in good shape and the set is about 20 or 30 years old.
    How many pieces are in the set? What is different about the top dresser drawers? What is the wood used in the set?

Directions: Listen to the information and answer the questions.

1. The first gallery you will pass through has paintings by American women. Beyond that, the gallery contains early American Indian artifacts. The next room has Amish quilts hanging on the walls. The last room to your left has antique jewelry, and the room beyond that on the right has a replica of a working blacksmith shop.
   Where does this take place? What is the third exhibit you will pass? What is in the second to last room?

2. Diane follows a predictable morning routine. She gets up, stretches for 10 minutes, then walks two miles. After she returns and takes a shower, she watches the news while she has coffee and a banana. She checks and refills the birdfeeder, answers her e-mail, does her hair, and gets dressed.
   What does Diane do while she watches the news? What does Diane do before she walks? What does she do right after she takes care of the birdfeeder?

3. The city-wide garage sale will take place in the North Oaks parking structure on Saturday. If you want to set up a table, you must reserve a space by Wednesday. Set-up starts at 6:00 A.M. on Saturday, but the public is not allowed inside until 8:00. Exhibitors are allowed to drive a vehicle inside the structure for set-up but it must be out of the structure by 7:30.
   If you want to participate in the garage sale, what do you have to do and when? When and where can you unload your car? When is the garage sale?

4. Tom was born in Albuquerque but is going to college in Florida now. His family was stationed in New Mexico while his father was in the Air Force. His father took a job in Chicago so the family moved when Tom was three. The family lived there until Tom graduated from high school.
   Where did the family live when Tom was born and why? Where did Tom spend most of his life? What is Tom doing now?

5. The police had searched all around the house and the neighbors' yards. While one officer got more information from the homeowner about the break-in, the other one radioed to send the sniffing dog. Twenty minutes later the dog arrived and was ready to work. In the meantime, one officer had found grass and mud in the kitchen that may have come off the burglar's shoe.
   How many officers were at the house? What was searched? Did the dog find anything?

6. We had a great time visiting London. When we got there we were exhausted, but right away we took a double-decker bus ride. Then we walked around Buckingham Palace. The next day we took a tour of the Victoria and Albert Museum that lasted the entire day. Before we left for Stonehenge, we got tickets and took a train to Windsor Castle for the day. We are exhausted but having a great time.
   What did the speaker do after the bus tour? What tour lasted all day? Where was the last place that we know the speaker went to?

7. After the introductory remarks, the first speaker will talk about relaxation techniques. There will be a 45-minute break during his talk for snacks and to visit the exhibit area of health supplements and exercise equipment. During that time attendees should also sign up for the free massages, yoga, and stretching classes that will occur in the afternoon. After the break, another speaker will talk about stress and diet after which you will have an hour for a healthy buffet lunch.
   What will the first speaker talk about? What happens after lunch? What two things can you do during the break?

8. Bud knew he would have at least two hours to wait while his wife got her hair cut and colored. He dropped off a watch to get a new battery installed, then he walked about a block to the bookstore. He bought a *Newsweek* and a *Wall Street Journal*. He saw a coffee shop and got coffee and a muffin and found an overstuffed chair in front of a coffee table. This wasn't so bad after all. He had picked up a bestseller list at the bookstore and checked it to see if any of the books appealed to him. He might get one to take home, but in the meantime he was content in his comfy chair.
   What is the first thing Bud did after leaving his wife? What will he probably do on the way back to pick her up? What has Bud bought so far?

9. We wanted to go to the park and walk around, but it was raining. We decided to try the mall, even though mall walking isn't good exercise for me because I do too much window shopping. We couldn't pass up all the smells at the food court so we stopped and had pizza. Then, we couldn't resist the Dollar Store—you never know what great deals you can find for a dollar. This was after we had already bought two pairs of shoes on sale.
   Why didn't the speakers go to the park? In what stores did they stop? What did they buy at the first place?

10. I don't think my father ever threw anything out. We expected to find a lot of old clothes in his closets, but we never expected to find boxes of old letters and cards from when he was growing up. Later we began to pull out all the old bottles in his medicine cabinet, and we noticed something lining one of the shelves. It looked like green shelf paper, but it was three $100 bills along the bottom of the middle shelf. We suddenly were more interested in the job. Then we went to his kitchen "junk" drawer by the sink. What do you think we found? A box in the back was filled with about 50 Susan B. Anthony silver dollars. Before we left we checked under his mattress and doormat, but no more surprises. We still have a huge attic full of stuff that we can look forward to sifting through.
    What was the first discovery? Where was the last place that was looked on the first day? Where were the silver dollars?

11. The inspector's report said the following should be done. The gutters are falling away from the house. They should be repaired with special gutter nails some time before winter. The roof will need to be replaced in about two years. Once the furniture has been moved in, it will be easier to see where to install recessed lighting and if the present electrical system will be adequate. The old oil furnace should be removed and a new gas forced-air furnace should be installed before anyone moves in.
    What is the first thing that should be done? When and how should the gutters be fixed? What needs to be checked in two years?

12. Erik's schedule for the next month involves a lot of travel. The first week he will be in Phoenix for a medical conference. While in the West, he will be attending a tax conference in San Diego. At the end of the month, he will attend two board meetings, one in New York City and then in Washington. After San Diego, he will fly to New York to give the keynote speech at the opening ceremony for a new science center at Cornell.
    What will he do in Phoenix? What is the last place he will go to and why? Where will he fly to from San Diego?

13. Chop one large onion, a small green pepper, and two stalks of celery into small pieces. Turn a burner to medium-high and put two tablespoons of butter and about one tablespoon of oil into a skillet. When the butter melts, add the vegetables. Let them cook while you set out a half-pound of Swiss cheese, four ounces chopped olives, ketchup, two chicken breasts, and two tablespoons of Cajun spices. When the vegetables are soft and have absorbed the oil, take them off the heat.
    What is the first thing you should do? What do you do after the butter melts? What do you think the recipe will make?

14. The drive to our place up north was not exactly as relaxing as we had hoped. We had driven about 45 minutes when we had to turn around because Wayne forgot to pack his pills. By the time we got back on the expressway there was more traffic, but it was moving along pretty well until we hit the construction. That really slowed us down, but we got to the outlet stores where we were stopping for lunch by 1:30. After eating and looking an hour for bargains, we started out again. An hour and a half later we switched to back roads where we enjoyed some much nicer scenery. We stopped at a roadside stand and got some homemade strawberry preserves, biscuits, and vegetables to take with us. We pulled in to the cottage around 6:00 which was just when the neighbors were also arriving.
    Why did they have a late lunch? What was the next place they stopped after lunch and how long did it take to get there? Why did Wayne have to go back home?

15. The class of 1999 reunion weekend starts with a kickoff rally on the quad Friday at 5:00. There will be drinks and snacks to enjoy while you catch up with old friends and make dinner plans. Dinner is on your own, but plan to be back at Noble Hall by 10:00 when the sounds of your alumni musicians, The Band Brats, will be reuniting and playing the oldies you enjoyed during your college days. Saturday and Sunday morning are class breakfasts at Lee Hall. Saturday morning at 10:00 you will gather with your class for the Alumni Parade. Saturday night's banquet is semi-formal. There are a number of sporting events and tours that are scheduled throughout the entire weekend, so be sure to leave time to take advantage of those.
    What would you miss if you did not arrive until Saturday at noon? What is the last planned event that is listed? When and where is the band playing?

16. The price is an all-encompassing $460. This includes a shuttle from the airport to the ship, three nights in a porthole room with a king-size bed and full bath, all meals, and all nonalcoholic beverages. It also includes seats for the first night's show spotlighting Broadway musicals and the last night's show with a celebrity comedian. It does not include airfare, alcoholic beverages, and tips. The ship features two deck pools, a casino, nightly entertainment, a spa, and a choice of four dining areas.
    What was described? What night does not include a show? What will you have to pay for?

17. The morning after graduating from University of Michigan, Amy and three of her pals got on a plane and headed to San Diego to take a relaxing cruise. A week after arriving home, she will again fly out, but this time to Ireland for a three-week seminar on British history. Amy has a four-week break before she will be moving into her new apartment in Pittsburgh. She will have two weeks to get settled before reporting to her fourth-grade teaching job. While at home, she will need to figure out what she will take, what supplies she will need for her classroom, and what she will buy in Pittsburgh for her new apartment.

    In between what two trips does Amy go to Ireland? Why is Amy moving? Where did Amy go right after graduation?

18. The meal was incredible. There were little baskets made of chocolate at each place. They were filled with chocolate truffles, cashews, and macadamias. As if that was not enough chocolate, there was a chocolate fountain at the dessert table which also had a variety of chocolate items. The first course was a chilled fruit soup—some sort of berry or combination of berries. There were also a few slices of melon on the salad of field greens, peppers, and onions that had a light, flavorful vinegar dressing. The breadbasket was delicious. There were three kinds of fresh, warm breads. The main course included a small filet mignon and a small piece of glazed salmon. There was a pile of little potatoes that had a yummy garlicky-buttery taste as well as a few spears of grilled asparagus on the plate.

    What was the dessert? What dishes included fruit? What was served on the dinner plate?

19. Patrick is waiting impatiently for responses to the 40 résumés he sent to human resource departments of companies in Boston. Patrick has come a long way from his first job right out of college with Microsoft. He stayed there for five years before he switched to Adobe as an assistant manager in the marketing department. There he realized that unless he got an MBA (master of business administration) he would never be able to get the kind of job that he really sought. He knew he liked spending more time with people and less with computers. So while he was at Adobe, he took evening classes and completed his MBA in four years.

    What are the companies on Patrick's résumé? When did he get his MBA? How long was Patrick at his first job?

20. Since I have the summer free, I am planning to divide my energies between the basement and outside. The first thing I want to do is sort through all the stuff in the basement and get rid of most of it. Then I want to divide the basement into an exercise room, an office, and a small room with floor-to-ceiling shelves. The basement cleanout will take the entire summer, so when I get bored with that, I will pull weeds, tend flowers, and prune bushes. I want to plant a small vegetable garden on the south side of the house at the beginning of the season and also plant some annuals in the backyard. However, I can't plant anything until those beds are dug out and the soil prepared.

    What will the speaker do after cleaning out the basement? What will the speaker do outside? What has to be done before planting the garden?

Directions: Listen to the information and answer the questions.

1. In the first three months of their lives, baby pelicans eat about 150 pounds of fish and may outweigh their parents. The baby birds need extra fat to survive during the time they are learning to fish for their own food. When the young birds leave the nest at about five weeks of age, they are often heavier than their parents.
   Why do the birds need fat? What is unusual about their weight? When do they leave the nest?

2. In Austin, Texas, two burglars broke into the home of Mr. and Mrs. David Conner. They stole two televisions and a checkbook. One of the burglars wrote a check made out to himself from the checkbook and took it to the local bank. When he showed it to the teller, the teller left and came back with a security guard. It turned out that the teller was Mrs. David Conner from the address where the men had stolen the checkbook.
   What did the burglars steal? Why was the teller suspicious? Where did this take place?

3. According to New York's *Daily News*, the world's most expensive omelet is on the menu at the Le Parker Meridien Hotel in New York City. The omelet is called "The Zillion Dollar Lobster Frittata" but it actually costs a thousand dollars. The creation is made with six eggs, lobster, and 10 ounces of sevruga caviar. The menu "dares you to expense this." Apparently, the dish is ordered, although not too often.
   Where is the item sold? How is it made? How much does it cost?

4. Some types of ants use the insect aphids like humans use cows. The ants protect the aphids and milk them like we milk cows. The tiny aphids suck sap from plants and produce a liquid called "honeydew." The ants eat and store the liquid for times when there is little food. To get the aphids to secrete the honeydew, ants stroke them with their antennae. Ants also will protect their aphids from ladybugs and other insects that prey on them.
   What is the liquid called that is produced by aphids? How do the ants get the liquid?
   What relationship are the ants and aphids compared to?

5. Mints do more than freshen your breath after a meal. Mints also help curb the buildup of gas in your stomach after you have ingested air during eating. Stomachs produce the gas buildup—it happens in everyone. The gas has to come out somehow, and we know what happens if it comes out in bursts. This is where mints are helpful. Peppermint contains natural oils that help the sphincter muscles to relax. When the sphincter relaxes, it allows gas to pass through it in a small steady stream that is quiet and unobtrusive.
   How does gas build up in the stomach? What are two uses of mints? What does peppermint contain and what does it do?

6. Some people have trouble getting to sleep. Some famous people had unusual ways of handling the problem. When Groucho Marx couldn't sleep, he would call people during the night and insult them. President Theodore Roosevelt took a shot of cognac in a glass of milk. W. C. Fields would stretch out on his billiards table and sleep there. When the poet Amy Lowell was traveling, she would rent five hotel rooms. She slept in one room, and rented the two rooms on either side, the room above, and the one below her sleeping room. She thought this would give her the complete quiet that she needed to get some rest.
   Who do you think had the strangest solution? Why did the poet rent five rooms? What would Groucho Marx do when he couldn't sleep?

7. The film *The Wizard of Oz* went through a number of changes before it was released. It was originally 120 minutes long but was shortened to 101 minutes. A dance number and some songs were cut. The "Over the Rainbow" song was almost cut because it made the Kansas scene too long and some thought it was degrading for Judy Garland to sing in a barnyard. The green horses in the City of Oz were colored with Jell-O crystals. The horse scenes had to be shot very quickly because the horses liked the flavor so much they kept licking it off. Judy Garland got very attached to Toto the dog and begged the owners to let her keep him, but they would not. Toto reportedly received $125 per week for his work.

   Why was the song almost cut? Why did the horse scene have to be shot quickly? How much did Toto earn?

8. Most people have heard of the Dutch boy who saved his country from flooding by putting his finger in the dike. For years, millions of tourists in the Netherlands have asked to see the place it happened. In 1950, the Dutch finally erected a memorial statue near Spaarndam Lock in memory of the boy and the dam. The interesting part is that, at first, the Dutch knew nothing about the finger in the dam story. That story was published in a fiction book called the *Silver Skates* by an American author. The Dutch people were approached so often about the boy and his brave deed that a statue was made to appease tourists and to create an attraction.

   Where did the deed actually happen? How did the statue help the tourist industry in Holland? When was the statue erected?

9. Mary Ann Smith was an elderly widow in Sydney, Australia, who liked gardening. One day she found a seedling growing in her garden coming up right where she had dumped a bunch of rotten apples. She decided to save the little tree, and she helped it grow. Eventually, it bore large green apples that had a tart flavor. Her neighbors liked them so much, they asked for cuttings from the tree so they could grow their own trees. When Mrs. Smith died in 1870, the green apple trees were thriving and they became known as Granny Smith's apples. By 1900, the apples were exported to the United States and are still known as Granny Smith apples.

   How were the apples described? How did the trees spread? What was the original name of the fruit?

10. Sylvan Goldman owned a chain of supermarkets in Oklahoma City. One day, he was inspired by two folding chairs in his office and he created the first shopping cart. On June 4, 1937, Goldman advertised his new invention as "the new innovation in shopping." However, it was not a big hit. Women said it reminded them of pushing a baby carriage, and men thought it was effeminate to push a cart. So Goldman decided to hire some male and female models of different ages to use the carts in the store. He had one employee handing out carts to the models and saying to women who weren't using one, "Everyone's using a cart, why aren't you?" It was the perfect gimmick. The cart idea took off. Mr. Goldman became a multimillionaire because he collected a royalty for every shopping cart bought in the United States until his patents ran out.

    How did Goldman come up with the idea? Why wasn't it popular at first? How did Goldman make his money?

11. "Handsome Dan" was a bulldog and the first official sports team mascot on record. In 1889, a Yale University student bought the bulldog for $5. The student dubbed him the Yale mascot. Handsome Dan accompanied his owner to Yale's sporting events who led him across the field on a leash before and after the football and baseball games. He barked at Yale successes and was intimidating to opponents. Yale students and faculty were so attached to the dog that when it died nine years later, the dog was stuffed and put in a trophy case. The original *Handsome Dan* remains on display in a sealed glass case in Yale's Payne Whitney Gymnasium. Ever since then, Yale has had a succession of Handsome Dan bulldogs as their mascot.

    When did the student get the original Handsome Dan and for how much? Where is the dog today? What university is this story about?

12. A gentleman was browsing at an Adamstown, Pennsylvania, flea market when he saw an old wooden picture frame with a country scene in it. He liked the frame and purchased the whole thing for $4. When he got home, he decided to remove the picture so he could use the frame. As he did, the frame fell apart and he found some folded paper between the canvas and wood backing of the frame. It turned out that the paper was an original 1776 copy of the Declaration of Independence. It was one of 500 official copies made from its first printing. The gentleman had Sotheby's Auction House sell it for him. On June 4, 1991, the document sold for $2,442,000. It was sold again in June 2000 for $8,140,000.

    How much did the man spend? What did he find? Why was it so valuable?

13. In 1997, Cathleen Byers had an unusual alibi for why she could not be found guilty of embezzlement. She worked for a credit union and admitted stealing $630,000 over a period of six years. However, she went on to say that she was not really guilty because she suffered from multiple personality disorder. She claimed that one of her other personalities must have been stealing but she had no knowledge of it at all. An expert on multiple personalities testified that the personality who stole the money didn't know right from wrong and that Ms. Byers would not have been aware of what her other personality was doing. However, Ms. Byers and her personalities were found guilty by a grand jury. The judge felt that Ms. Byers was guilty and he argued that even if another personality committed the crime she "should have been clued in by her new house and the luxury cars."

    How much did Byers steal? Why did she feel she should not be found guilty? Who do you agree with and why?

14. Jason Powell was working on a large farm in Oregon in 2002. The farm raised grasses that were sold commercially around the world. One day after he finished working in a field, Jason reached for his wallet and couldn't find it. He figured it had fallen out of his pocket somewhere in the field. Jason had no idea that his wallet had been picked up in a large combine that was cutting grass to make hay bales. The wallet was inside one of the bales. This bale along with many others was sent to a farmer in Japan who had purchased them to feed his animals. One day when the farmer was breaking apart the bale to feed his cattle, the wallet fell out. When he checked it, he found identification and decided to send it back to its owner. Jason received his wallet totally intact with his driver's license, credit cards, and six one-dollar bills about half a year after he lost it.

    What kind of farm was Jason working on? Explain how the wallet got to Japan. What was in the wallet?

15. Copper is used on the bottom of pots and pans for more than decorative reasons. Copper-bottomed utensils distribute heat over the entire bottom of the pot so that the food will cook more evenly. Early cowboys wearing Levi jeans found out about copper's benefits the hard way. Before 1942, all Levi 501 jeans had copper rivets in six places. One of those places was where the main seams of the legs came together. Legend, and an old Levis commercial, has it that as the cowboys sat in front of the campfire, the rivets got very warm and stayed warm for a while. That was rather uncomfortable for the cowboys, but it also proved what a great conductor of heat copper is.
    Why is copper used in pots and pans? When were the copper rivets changed? What does the story prove about copper?

16. In 2000, David Phillips collected enough bar codes from Healthy Choice pudding cups to earn 1,253,000 free frequent flyer miles. Mr. Phillips read about a Healthy Choice promotion in which he could earn 500 frequent flyer miles by sending in 10 bar codes from Healthy Choice products by a certain date. Through looking around, he found individual pudding cups that he could buy for a quarter each. He bought more than 12,000 individual puddings. He realized he could not remove the bar codes by himself to meet the deadline, so he came up with a plan. He donated the pudding to a food bank and the Salvation Army with the agreement that they would tear off each bar code and give it back to him. They happily complied and were happy to get the pudding. David began making packets of bar codes. Ten bar codes got him a certificate for 500 miles. Soon he began receiving certificates from Healthy Choice. David got at least two additional perks from the promotion. Because he banked over one million miles with American Airlines, he was given a life membership into the exclusive Advantage Gold membership Club. And since David had donated all that pudding to charitable organizations, he was able to take a tax write-off of $815.
    What was the deal that got David started? How much pudding did he buy? What else did David end up receiving?

17. Is there really a basketball court inside the top of the Matterhorn roller coaster at Disneyland? According to legend, Anaheim had a height ordinance that applied to all structures except sports facilities. The court was built into the Mountain so it could be considered a sports arena and therefore be built as high as Disney needed it. That made a good story, but the truth is this: There is an area built inside the top of Matterhorn Mountain that is about the size of a half-court and does have a basketball hoop in it. It was intended as an area for climbers who sometimes scaled the mountain to entertain Disney guests. This area gave them a place to rest and pass the time when they weren't performing or the weather was bad.
    What is the legend about the basketball court? What is the area used for? Why do people climb the mountain?

18. The line "I don't get no respect" was made famous by comedian Rodney Dangerfield. In an interview in 2004 on National Public Radio, Rodney explained how the line started. When the *Godfather* movie came out in 1972, the Godfather says about a woman, "When she's with me, you show her respect . . . I want respect." That line about showing respect became very popular. Dangerfield decided to write a joke with a variation of the Godfather line. He said this was the first joke he ever wrote. The joke was, "I don't get no respect. When I was a kid, my friends played hide-and-seek. They wouldn't even look for me, you know." Rodney Dangerfield then added in the interview, "And all of a sudden, I found an image." Dangerfield died soon after that interview, but the line "I don't get no respect" will remain as his forever.
    Where did the line come from? What was Rodney's first joke? When was the interview?

19. The Tinker & Partners advertising firm created a great marketing gimmick for Alka-Seltzer in the 1960s. They changed the focus of Alka-Seltzer ads from pain to pleasure. The new ads showed a series of amusing stomachs such as the bouncing stomach of a man using a jackhammer. They produced a series of upbeat commercials. One of them had a "cocktail" of Alka-Seltzer on the rocks showing two tablets plopping into a crystal glass of water. Up until that time, the directions were to put one tablet in water. New directions on the package were changed to put two tablets in water, and soon small foil-wrapped packages with two tablets in them were packaged. This change to cute, positive ads and the suggestion to use two tablets instead of one almost doubled the sales of the product. The phrase "pop, pop, fizz, fizz" came a little later and remains in people's minds today when they think of Alka-Seltzer.

    What did the 1960s ads show? Why was the cocktail a good ad? What was probably the main thing that increased sales?

20. There are some interesting facts about the Hershey's Kiss candies. It was originally named for the sound and motion of the machine that produced it. When the chocolate was extruded from the machine onto the conveyor belt it looked like the machine was kissing the belt and it also made a noise like a kiss. In Hershey, Pennsylvania, the street lamps are shaped like Kisses. It takes 99 Kisses to make one pound of chocolate. A machine started wrapping the candies in foil in 1921, and the tiny flag saying "Hershey's" was added to ensure the product was the real thing. Imitators were cropping up, and so the flag, or "plume" as it is officially called, was registered as a trademark in 1924. From 1942 to 1949, the production of Kisses was stopped in order to save foil during World War II. During that time, Hershey's mixers prepared chocolate military rations for soldiers.

    How did the candy get its name? When was production stopped on the candy and why? What is the official name of the flag with Hershey's on it and when was it trademarked?

Directions: Each item has a conversation between two or occasionally three speakers. Listen and answer the questions that follow.

1. **A**: Do you come here often? **B**: No, it's my first time. I came with a friend who is a regular. **A**: Can I buy you a drink? **B**: No thanks, we're waiting for a table and we could be called any minute. **A**: Come by after you eat. I'll still be here and I'd like to get to know you.
   Where does this take place? Why does the person turn down the drink offer?

2. **A**: How can I help you? **B**: I would like to send this Priority Mail. **A**: That will be $16.95. Do you want insurance for it? **B**: How much more would that be? Oh, and while I'm here, I'll take a book of stamps. **A**: The cost depends on how much insurance you want. A book of 20 stamps is $7.80.
   Where is this conversation taking place? What do you know the person will be paying for?

3. **A**: He painted with rich colors that impart a sense of serenity and passion at the same time. **B**: How much is it? **A**: It's an original and the last one in this series of bold colors before the artist switched to pen and ink. **B**: How much? **A:** $4,500.
   What are the speakers discussing? What is the artist doing now?

4. **A**: She's here! It's a girl and she was born at 10:13 P.M. **B**: Congratulations! How's Janie doing and have you decided on a name? **A**: Well, it will be either Heather or Megan or Samantha. Her middle name will be Doyle. **B**: I really like Samantha. What did she weigh? **A**: She was 6 pounds, 12 ounces and is 18 inches long.
   What question did the father not answer? What name has been decided and what is it?

5. **A**: Matt, we heard about your opponent. Now tell us about what you do. **B**: I started the A-B-C Fitness Centers. **A**: Where are they located? **B**: We have four in Iowa and I'm opening two more this year. **B**: That's great. What does A-B-C stand for? **A**: I'm glad you asked. It stands for abs, buns, and cardio—the three areas everyone wants to improve, and that's what we work on.
   What are the speakers discussing and where are they probably talking? What do the company's initials stand for?

6. **A**: Mrs. Wood is so unfair. She must think we have nothing else to do with our lives. **B**: Yeah, how am I supposed to read two chapters, do my math, go to soccer, and watch *American Idol*? There's no way. **A**: I have to stay on the honor roll so I've got to—and at least the only other thing you have is math. I have to write an eight-line poem too. **B**: You ought to write about how we get too much homework. **A**: Great idea!
   Who are the speakers and what are they discussing? What is the assignment?

7. **A**: What are the results? **B**: It's a cyst and it should go away by itself. There is no sign of malignancy. **A**: So, do I need to do anything else? **B**: No, you are all set. However, if you feel it getting bigger or notice any other changes, make an appointment. **A**: Thanks, that's a big relief.
   Who are the speakers and what are they discussing? What is the next step?

8. **A**: I've checked the pipes out of here and they are pretty clear. I think the problem is between your house and the connection to the main sewer line. **B**: Why would there be a problem there? **A**: We get a lot of calls in this area, and usually it turns out to be tree limbs that have grown into the pipe. Things going through your line can get caught on even a tiny twig and cause a plug that can back up. **B**: So what do you suggest? **A**: The whole area should be snaked to open up the pipes and pull out any debris that is clogging them.
   Who are the speakers? What is the likely cause of the problem?

9. **A**: Our party special includes two appetizers, two salads, broasted chicken, and lasagna. It also includes plastic serving pieces and napkins. Plastic utensils and plates are extra. We only charge $10 to deliver it. **B**: How much would that run for 15 people? **A**: The special feeds 12 and it is $85. It might feed 15 depending on how hungry they are. Or we can add a charge of $9.95 per person for three more people. **B**: You didn't say anything about bread or rolls. **A**: Oh, sorry. It does include our soft garlic breadsticks.
   What are the speakers discussing? Name all the food items that are included.

10. **A**: Welcome, folks, to the opening game of the Eastern Division NBA Playoffs. **B**: This is going to be a great game with both teams pretty evenly matched and pumped up for a big win. **A**: These teams have faced each other in postseason twice, and they split the games. Can't get much more even than that. **B**: We have word that veteran forward Terry Wallace will not play in game one because of back spasms. **A**: That's a good move because they will need him totally rested and ready to give it all in game two.
    Who are the speakers and where are they? What sport are they discussing?

11. **A**: This situation is out of control. I know you think you are being a good parent, but you have got to get real. Buying your kid whatever he wants so he won't throw a fit is not a solution. **B**: I know I shouldn't give in, but I want him to have the things I didn't have. **A**: You need to read my book on parenting. And you need to take a good look at what you are creating. Part of being a parent is teaching your child that life is not always fair and how to cope with disappointment. How is he learning to cope when he never has any disappointment? **B**: Well, I just want him to be happy.
    Who are the speakers? What is the parent doing wrong?

12. **A**: Why did you leave your current job? **B**: I learned a lot in my seven years at Ames, but I am interested in a position in which I can expand my creative abilities. **A**: We are looking for creativity but also a solid background in computer graphics and design. What experience do you have that melds the two? **B**: In my last job I wrote and designed all of the promotional materials. These were all computer-generated. I have brought samples of my work in that area. **A**: Good. I would like to see them.
    What is the situation and who are the speakers? What question was not answered?

13. **A**: You asked me to call you if Maddy was pregnant. She is very pregnant; the litter is due in four weeks. **B**: Who was she bred with? **A**: His name is Cooper. Check my website and you can see pictures of them. **B**: I know Maddy, but what is Cooper like? **A**: Cooper is a sweetheart. He is lighter in color and a bit heavier than Maddy. He is very laid-back and loves chasing balls. He has not been shown but has competed in agility trials.
    What are the speakers talking about? Describe the father.

14. **A**: Good evening, Miss Virginia. Where are you from? **B**: I'm from the little town of Oakville, home of the largest working windmill in the country and the best corn dogs in the world. **A**: What will you promote during your reign if you win? **B**: My platform is about dental hygiene. Most people do not know what a critical part clean teeth play in giving you a healthy and happy life. **A**: Thank you, Miss Virginia. I am sure you have the support of all America's dentists.
 Where did this conversation take place? What is special about her hometown?

15. **A**: You have insurance for your car. Isn't your life more important than your car? **B**: Of course, but I can't afford another payment right now. **A**: Can you afford a dollar a day? Your daily coffee costs more than that. **B**: I'll think about it. **A**: You can't afford to just think about it. These super-low rates are because you are young and healthy. If you sign up today, I will also give you this *Entertainment* coupon book so you can save even more money all year.
 What is the conversation about? What would you say in response?

16. **A**: I'm sorry but this is just not working for me. **B**: What do you mean? **A**: It's not you—it's just that I'm not in a place in my life where I want to get serious with anyone. **B**: And what have we been doing the past year? **A**: We've had a great time and I'll always remember that. But it's time for me to move on. I really need to concentrate on my work.
 What is the conversation about? How would you handle the conversation?

17. **A**: When I was a boy, we didn't have computers, and all the phones were tied to a line in the wall. **B**: Boring. **A**: We actually played with toys and games. Real games—not the video kind. **B**: Like what? **A**: We had pick-up ball games, hula hoops. We rode bikes everywhere and we played games like Clue and Monopoly and Chinese Checkers. **B**: Boring.
 What is the conversation about? About how old would you guess the speakers are?

18. **A**: We can't guarantee this rate when you are ready to close unless you lock it in today. **B**: Has the market fluctuated a lot in the past couple of months? **A**: Market indicators are that interest rates are on a slow increase. They could go up at any time. **B**: How long do I have to make the decision? **A**: You have four business days to guarantee this rate.
 What are the speakers discussing? What would you do in the situation?

19. **A**: The question I pose to both candidates is: What is your plan for bringing more jobs to the state? **B**: We are a very desirable state for new and expanding businesses. We have resources, climate, opportunity, a low business tax, and we will continue to meet with major companies and show them the advantages of our state. **C**: We need to do much more to bring jobs to this state. We have an extensive plan for companies that includes tax breaks, major highway and airport access, and other governmental incentives. In addition, we intend to make this state the first all-wireless one in the country. That would be a major draw for small and large businesses. **A**: I have a follow-up question regarding the current small-business tax.
 Who are the three speakers? Which candidate will businesses like and why?

20. **A**: It's the emerald ash borer, all right. Sorry, but that tree will have to go before it will or already has infected more trees. **B**: What do we have to do? **A**: There are companies that deal with this and you will have to get in touch with them. Try your city hall. This is a quarantined area and anyone who takes an ash down has to follow a bunch of special rules. **B**: How much will all this cost? **A**: I don't know, but you can bet it will be more because of those regulations and the special disposal.
 What is the problem? Why does a special company need to be called?

Directions: Listen to the information and answer the questions.

1. This is a list of common things with uncommon names. A snorkel box is a roadside mailbox with the opening under a curved top that you can use without leaving your car. A heeltap is the tiny bit of liquid left in a glass after you have finished an alcoholic drink. The grumbling sound of an upset stomach is called wamble. The holder that is put around paper cups that contain hot liquids is a zarf. The lunula is the small white half-moon part of your nails.
   What is wamble? What is the white half-moon part of your nails called? Where do you find a heeltap?

2. This is a list of interesting skills. The record for stacking dominoes vertically is 726 dominoes high. The fastest time to shear one sheep is 45.41 seconds. The longest distance that a grape was thrown and caught in the mouth is 327 feet, 6 inches. The most books balanced on a person's head is 62. The record for the most yo-yo tricks done in one minute is 51.
   Which record do you think is the most impressive? What happened in less than one minute? How many dominoes were stacked up?

3. This is a list of activities and their times. The community center will host a newcomer's tea on Tuesday morning at 11:00. Wednesday at 9:00, the fiction book club meets, and at 2:00 the biography book club will meet. There is a Bingo game Thursday evenings at 7:00. Friday morning at 8:00 is aerobics, and yoga is at 9:30.
   If you like to read, what day's activities would you be interested in? What type of exercise is in the earlier class? What is scheduled Tuesday at 11:00?

4. This is a list of some of the things your body does in one day. Your body sheds 36 million skin cells. Your heart beats 100,800 times. Ten billion white blood cells are made every day. You shed 40 to 100 strands of hair daily. One teaspoon of tears falls from your eyes.
   What is made every day in the body? How many cells are shed and what type are they? What do you produce that could fill a teaspoon?

5. This is a list of people and movies that were made about them. *Finding Neverland* is about J. M. Barrie who wrote *Peter Pan. What's Love Got to Do with It* is about Tina Turner. *8 Seconds* is about rodeo champion Lane Frost. *Immortal Beloved* is the story of Ludwig Van Beethoven. *Walk the Line* is the story of Johnny Cash.
   Which movies are about musicians? Which one is about an author? What is the name of the movie about the rodeo?

6. This is a list of some Academy Award Best Pictures and their stars. *Casablanca* with Humphrey Bogart and Ingrid Bergman won in 1942. In 1951 *An American in Paris* with Gene Kelly and Leslie Caron won. *Out of Africa* starring Robert Redford and Meryl Streep won in 1985. In 1990 *Dances with Wolves* with Kevin Costner won. *Unforgiven* with Clint Eastwood and Gene Hackman won in 1992.
   What are the five pictures that won? What were the two that won in the 1990s? Who did Ingrid Bergman star with?

7. This is a list of people and their responsibilities for the fundraiser. Cindy will work directly with the speaker. Charley is responsible for the flyer. Carol will compile a mailing list. Katy will contact and secure sponsors. Cory will put together the specific program, and Kim will oversee the entire event.
   What do all the names have in common? Who will contact the speaker? How many different jobs are listed?

8. This is a list of "lasts." The last play that Shakespeare wrote was *The Tempest* in 1611. The last Beatles concert was in San Francisco in 1966. The last cigarette ad on TV was in 1970. The last dodo bird died in 168 1. The last year that quarters and dimes actually had silver in them was 1964.
   Which "last" affected you the most? Which two things happened closest together? What does silver have to do with this list?

9. According to legend, there are a number of ways to protect yourself from a vampire. Draping fishnet and knotted string around doorways is supposed to keep vampires out because they will want to untangle them. Mirrors on doors keep them away because vampires are frustrated that they can't see their own reflections. If you leave branches of a holly or juniper tree on the floor, vampires will trip over them. Wearing garlic cloves around your neck should keep vampires away. Vampires hate water, so always carry a big water bottle with you.
   What is the easiest way to keep vampires away and why? What type of branch will vampires trip over? What do you do around doorways and why?

10. This is a list of inventors and their patented inventions. Jacob Schick invented the electric razor. Clarence Birdseye invented packaged frozen foods. Walter Hunt invented the safety pin. Mark Twain invented suspenders. John Rand invented the toothpaste tube. Chester Greenwood invented earmuffs.
    Who invented the clothing? Which two inventors' names are still on the product today? What did John Rand invent?

11. This is a list of television firsts. The first TV commercial was a 10-second ad for a Bulova clock in 1941. The first broadcast of *Meet the Press* was in 1947. This show is also the longest-running show on TV. The first president to appear on TV was Franklin D. Roosevelt in 1939 when he opened the New York World's Fair. The first soap opera on television was *A Woman to Remember* that started on radio and moved to TV in 1949. The first nationwide color broadcast was the Tournament of Roses parade on January 1, 1954.
    What is the longest-running show and when did it start? Why did the president first appear on television? About how long has the Tournament of Roses parade been on TV?

12. This is a list of unusual museums. The Cockroach Hall of Fame in Texas has insects dressed as famous people. You can visit the Baked Bean Museum of Excellence in Wales and see over 200 baked bean memorabilia and exhibits. The Museum of Dirt in Massachusetts has more than 300 samples of dirt from around the world. The Lunchbox Museum in Georgia has more than 2,000 metal lunchboxes. At the Museum of Spam in Minnesota, you will learn everything you could possibly know about Hormel Spam. The Barney Smith's Toilet Seat Art Museum in Texas has over 700 decorated toilet seats.
    What are the names of the museums? Which museum do you think is the weirdest? Which one has 700 items on display?

13. This is a list of unusual animal facts. An ostrich's eye is bigger than its brain. Cats have 32 muscles in each ear. Tigers have striped skin in addition to striped fur. A beaver's teeth never stop growing. A pig is the only animal that can get sunburned. A woodchuck only breathes 10 times during its hibernation.
    What is unusual about tigers? Which animal has an unusual hibernation? Which one has the smallest brain?

14. This is a list of short tongue twisters. Three tree twigs. Yellow linoleum. Chopped chocolate chips. Six thick sticks. Black bugs blood. Fresh fried fish.
    Repeat each of them three times. Can you think of a three-word tongue twister? What was the third one?

15. This is a list of strange laws. It is illegal to sing off-key in North Carolina. In Massachusetts, mourners at a wake may not eat more than three sandwiches. In Canada, it is illegal to pay off a debt higher than 25 cents in pennies. In Kansas, it is illegal to shoot rabbits from a motorboat. It is illegal to play dominoes on Sunday in Alabama. You cannot run for governor of Pennsylvania if you have ever been in a duel.
    Which law is not from a state and what is it? What states were mentioned? If you don't sing well, where could you be arrested?

16. This is a list of places that don't live up to their names. Buenos Aires means "good winds" but only because early sailors prayed for good winds before venturing out. Singapore means "City of Lions," but lions don't live there. Greenland is not green; it is white from ice. Nome, Alaska, got its name from someone misreading the word *name*. Pacific Ocean is from *Mar Pacifico* meaning *calm sea*, except that the Pacific has very stormy seas. The story of the name Yucatan is that a Spanish explorer asked a native the name of the peninsula and he replied "Yukatan" which to the native meant "I don't understand you."
    What means "City of Lions?" What did Yucatan mean to the natives? How was the city in Alaska named?

17. This is a list of facts about your body. If all the blood vessels in your body were laid end to end, they would reach 60,000 miles. Each person has a unique tongue print. It takes 17 muscles to smile and 43 muscles to frown. The left lung is smaller than the right lung because it has to make room for the heart. The most common blood type is O, and the rarest is type A-H. There are 45 miles of nerves in the body.
    What is the rarest blood type? If you laid them end to end, would your nerves or your blood vessels be longer? Which lung is smaller and why?

18. This is a list of weather records. The largest variation in temperature in 24 hours was 100° in Browning, Montana, in 1916. In 1959, the Mount Shasta Ski Bowl in California recorded a record 189 inches of snow that fell during one snowstorm. The heaviest hailstone recorded weighed 2.25 pounds and fell in Bangladesh in 1986. The lowest temperature ever recorded was negative 128.6° Fahrenheit in Antarctica in 1983. The highest temperature was 134° Fahrenheit and was recorded in Death Valley, California, in 1913.
    Where was the heaviest hailstone? Where was the greatest temperature variation and what was the variation? What were the events that happened in California?

19. This is a list of words that are not what they appear to be. Koala bears are not bears; they are marsupials. Fireflies are not flies; they are beetles. Guinea pigs are not from Guinea and they are not pigs; they are rodents from South America. Wild rice is not wild or a rice; it is a harvested crop in the grass family. Butterflies have nothing to do with butter and are not flies; they are related to the moth. Grape-Nuts cereal has neither grapes nor nuts in it; it was named because a grape-like sugar is formed during the cooking process and the cereal has a nutty flavor. The funny bone is not funny and not a bone. It is a nerve.

    What is similar about koala bears and guinea pigs? What is the fourth item? Explain about the name of the cereal.

20. This is a list of what it means if you dream about milk. If you dream about milk in large containers, it means you will have riches and honor. If you dream that you are in the milk business as in buying and selling it, the dream means you will be successful in life. If you dream that you give milk away, it means you are too generous and could have financial problems. If you dream of spilling milk, it means your friends will disappoint you. If you dream about spoiled milk, it means you will have many little frustrations. If you dream you are trying to drink milk but cannot swallow it, it means you may be losing a long-time friend.

    What kind of dream means your friends will disappoint you? What does dreaming about spoiled milk mean? If you think that dreams come true, which dream would you like to have about milk?

NONVERBAL COMMUNICATION

Directions: Use gestures to show the following concepts.

1. yes
2. no
3. I can't hear you
4. I don't know
5. (point to) something you want
6. OK
7. I don't care
8. go away
9. (there was a call or to call someone) telephone
10. (television or radio) turn it on
11. take a shower
12. go for a walk
13. come over here
14. what's wrong
15. I don't understand
16. thank you
17. (I am in) pain
18. I don't want to
19. Where is the remote control?
20. (repeat what you said) say it again

Directions: Use gestures to get across the idea.

1. I need to go to the bathroom.
2. I don't feel well.
3. I am hungry.
4. I am thirsty.
5. I want to exercise.
6. I am upset.
7. I am angry.
8. I am hot.
9. I am cold.
10. When are you coming back?
11. I have a headache.
12. My stomach hurts.
13. I am tired.
14. I want to see my doctor.
15. I want the paper.
16. Turn off the light.
17. Please be quiet.
18. What time is it?
19. I want to go to bed.
20. I need my glasses.

Directions: Use gestures to indicate the word and then show the opposite of the word.

1. happy and ________
2. left and ________
3. black and ________
4. in and ________
5. first and ________
6. stop and ________
7. front and ________
8. fat and ________
9. up and ________
10. hot and ________
11. yes and ________
12. north and ________
13. fast and ________
14. long and ________
15. over and ________
16. cry and ________
17. on and ________
18. big and ________
19. open and ________
20. good and ________

Directions: Use gestures to answer the question.

Show how you would . . .

1. use a fork to eat
2. use a file on your nails
3. use your arms to swim
4. use barbells to exercise
5. wear a scarf to keep warm
6. use a cane to help you walk
7. use a match to light a candle
8. play a harmonica
9. hold a pen to write your name
10. use a razor to shave
11. hold a glass to make a toast
12. use a key to open a door
13. use a ruler to measure this book
14. use a straw to drink
15. use a towel to dry your hair
16. throw a Frisbee
17. use a sponge to wipe up a spill
18. answer a phone
19. use cologne
20. roll a bowling ball

Directions: Use nonverbal means to answer the question.

1. How do you act when you are angry?
2. How do you get someone's attention?
3. How do you eat a hot dog?
4. How would you act if you were bored?
5. How do you blow a kiss?
6. How do you use a magnifying glass?
7. How do you use a steering wheel?
8. How do you use a microphone?
9. How does a rabbit move?
10. How do you act surprised?
11. How do you flip pancakes?
12. What does poison ivy make you do?
13. What do people do under mistletoe?
14. How do you use a shoehorn?
15. How do you use a punching bag?
16. How do you move in a wheelchair?
17. Where do people have dandruff?
18. How do people show off their biceps?
19. What do you do when you get a cramp?
20. How do you play soccer?

Pantomime

Directions: Use gestures to show the idea.

1. pouring a drink
2. playing a piano
3. combing your hair
4. swatting a fly
5. ringing a bell
6. petting an animal
7. casting a fishing line
8. hitting a baseball
9. blowing your nose
10. applauding a performer
11. putting on lipstick / shaving
12. signaling for a bus to stop
13. opening a window
14. taking your pulse
15. washing your hands
16. stretching when you wake up
17. painting a wall
18. smelling a rose
19. bouncing a ball
20. rocking a baby

Directions: Use gestures to show the idea.

1. shaking hands
2. sneezing
3. falling or losing your balance
4. drinking
5. pouting
6. whispering
7. gargling
8. chewing
9. crying
10. sitting down
11. stay away
12. saluting
13. hiccuping
14. shivering
15. choking
16. panting
17. blushing
18. laughing
19. sleeping
20. hugging

Show Function

Directions: Use gestures to demonstrate how to use each item.

Show me what you do with . . .

1. a handkerchief
2. a banana
3. deodorant
4. dice
5. drums
6. earrings
7. a mirror
8. pills
9. a faucet
10. mouthwash
11. a seat belt
12. an umbrella
13. a rolling pin
14. a belt
15. a suitcase
16. a sandwich
17. binoculars
18. a slot machine
19. a saw
20. a basketball

Directions: Use nonverbal means to show you understand the meaning of the word.

1. pillow
2. scissors
3. hips
4. toothbrush
5. pencil
6. skunk
7. sleeves
8. newspaper
9. drums
10. body cream / lotion
11. heart
12. bell
13. thumb
14. rooster
15. hearing aid
16. poison
17. wedding ring
18. stairs
19. wig
20. dentures

Drawing

Directions: Draw the items.

1. dollar bill
2. phone
3. bottle
4. plate of food
5. television
6. cup or mug
7. frying pan
8. button
9. stick figure
10. house
11. smiley face
12. shoe
13. lips
14. cane
15. book
16. envelope
17. bed
18. chair
19. cat or dog
20. compass

Directions: Draw what is described.

1. What do you use to tell time?
2. What do you use to cut meat?
3. What do you use to write?
4. What does a bouquet contain?
5. What do you drink water or juice from?
6. What is a fruit that is cut up and baked in pies?
7. What is worn around the neck with a shirt?
8. What do you go through to enter your home?
9. What lands at an airport?
10. What can you see in the sky at night?
11. What do you wear on your hands when they are cold?
12. What do you wear on your eyes to help you see?
13. What is the bottom part of a suit?
14. What do you use to sweep a floor?
15. What does a chicken lay?
16. What do you use to clean your teeth?
17. What do you turn on to provide light?
18. What do you use to pound nails into a wall?
19. What provides shade from the heat of the sun?
20. What burns in a fireplace?

Draw in a Category

Directions: Draw one or more items that fit in the category.

1. clothing
2. parts of your body
3. fruits
4. shapes
5. money
6. sports
7. desserts
8. things used to clean a house
9. items used to set a table
10. jewelry
11. animals smaller than a pony
12. breakfast foods
13. flowers
14. weather conditions
15. grooming supplies
16. tools in a toolbox
17. items in or on a desk
18. things found in a kitchen
19. things found in a living room
20. things found in a garage

Directions: Use nonverbal means to answer the question.

1. Where does it hurt if you have laryngitis?
2. How many things are in a dozen?
3. How do you play a guitar?
4. What is used to fire a bullet?
5. How do you zip up a jacket?
6. When was the last time it rained?
7. Where is your lap?
8. Where could you have a pimple?
9. What time does it get dark outside?
10. How does a conductor lead an orchestra?
11. What symbol is associated with Valentine's Day?
12. How do you eat an ice cream cone?
13. What is dandruff?
14. What is the size and shape of a watermelon?
15. How do you light and extinguish a candle?
16. How do babies get around before they walk?
17. What do you do with bubble gum?
18. How can you tell that a woman is pregnant?
19. Where would you find a bald spot?
20. How do you eat corn on the cob?

Personal Questions

Directions: Use nonverbal means to answer the question.

1. In what month is your birthday?
2. When did you get up this morning?
3. When do you go to bed at night?
4. What state do you live in?
5. How many brothers or sisters do you have?
6. Where do you carry your money?
7. What do you usually have for breakfast?
8. Who do you live with?
9. When was the last time you ate?
10. What are you going to do after you finish these questions?
11. What do you have in your pockets?
12. What do you worry about?
13. What do you like to drink?
14. What do you do for exercise?
15. What day of the week is it?
16. What is something you really like to eat?
17. How many children do you have?
18. What is your favorite color?
19. When did you graduate from high school?
20. What is something you enjoy doing?

Directions: Use nonverbal means to answer the question.

1. What sport do you enjoy watching?
2. What did you do last weekend?
3. What is a special talent you or someone in your family has?
4. Where do you like to go for a dinner out?
5. What type of home do you live in?
6. What is the weather forecast for tonight?
7. What kind of vacation do you like to take?
8. In what state were you born?
9. What do you think is a big problem in America?
10. What kind of car does your family have?
11. What do you like to watch on TV?
12. Draw a plan of the main floor of your home.
13. Show me the route you take from home to here (or to some other specific place).
14. What is something you really liked doing when you were younger?
15. What household chore do you not like doing?
16. What do you like to do on a weekend?
17. Most people have a specialty food they like to cook. What is yours?
18. If you won the lottery, what is a big splurge item you would buy?
19. What place do you enjoy visiting again and again?
20. What type of music do you like to listen to?

COMPLETIONS

Directions: Common functional phrases are given with the final word missing. The completion word should be appropriate to the individual. Some possible words are suggested in parentheses.

1. How are _________
2. I feel _________ (fine, great, lousy, OK)
3. Have a nice _________
4. Thank _________
5. See you _________ (later)
6. Take a _________ (shower, ride, nap)
7. I want to go _________ (home, store, car, out, bed)
8. I need _________ (bathroom, doctor, help)
9. I love _________
10. O- _________ (OK)
11. I want _________ (food, water, more, paper, you)
12. Where are you _________ (going, from)
13. Go for a _________ (walk, ride)
14. I don't feel _________ (well, good, right)
15. I want to _________ (sleep, walk, exercise, eat, go, wash)
16. Turn on the _________ (TV, light, radio)
17. I'm _________ (hungry, thirsty, tired)
18. I want the _________ (paper, mail)
19. I'm too _________ (hot, cold, sick)
20. Answer the _________ (phone, door)

Directions: Complete the sentence with a word (or words) that makes sense.

1. Sing a _________
2. Clap your _________
3. Button your _________
4. Iron the _________
5. Comb your _________
6. Cash a _________
7. Brush your _________
8. Mow the _________
9. Spend your _________
10. Open the _________
11. Drive a _________
12. Answer the _________
13. Blink your _________
14. Dig a _________
15. Park the _________
16. Water the _________
17. Climb the _________
18. Write a _________
19. Flush the _________
20. Pay the _________

Directions: Complete the phrase with the opposite of the first word.

1. yes and _________
2. happy and _________
3. wet and _________
4. young and _________
5. long and _________
6. easy and _________
7. in and _________
8. day and _________
9. before and _________
10. hot and _________
11. good and _________
12. stop and _________
13. off and _________
14. left and _________
15. big and _________
16. hello and _________
17. fast and _________
18. up and _________
19. open and _________
20. laugh and _________

Directions: Complete the phrase with a word that goes with the first one.

1. brush and __________
2. table and __________
3. bread and __________
4. thunder and __________
5. knife and __________
6. shoes and __________
7. hugs and __________
8. soap and __________
9. sunny and __________
10. brother and __________
11. salt and __________
12. shirt and __________
13. winter and __________
14. read and __________
15. aunt and __________
16. dogs and __________
17. lightning and __________
18. pen and __________
19. washer and __________
20. ladies and __________

Directions: Complete the name of the food.

1. macaroni and _________
2. peanut butter and _________
3. corn on the _________
4. French fried _________
5. chicken noodle _________
6. pepperoni and cheese _________
7. corned beef and _________
8. banana cream _________
9. a glass of skim _________
10. eggs and _________
11. a chocolate chip _________
12. a hot dog on a _________
13. a grilled cheese _________
14. a hot fudge _________
15. turkey and _________
16. a hard-boiled _________
17. a glass of orange _________
18. a medium decaf _________
19. a bowl of vanilla _________
20. New England clam _________

Expressions

Directions: Complete the sentence by adding the last word of the expression.

1. The check is in the _________
2. A chip off the old _________
3. He's got ants in his _________
4. No pain, no _________
5. Sign on the dotted _________
6. In the twinkling of an _________
7. Make up for lost _________
8. It's on the tip of my _________
9. Three strikes and you're _________
10. Better late than _________
11. Read between the _________
12. Stick out your _________
13. Keep a stiff upper _________
14. Take one step at a _________
15. There's no place like _________
16. Don't drink and _________
17. The calm before the _________
18. It was love at first _________
19. The squeaky wheel gets the _________
20. A big fish in a little _________

Directions: Complete the saying with the word that is missing.

1. What goes up must come _________
2. Actions speak louder than _________
3. Don't call us, we'll call _________
4. Practice what you _________
5. It's easier said than _________
6. His bark is worse than his _________
7. What you see is what you _________
8. Absence makes the heart grow _________
9. Save it for a rainy _________
10. Do as I say, not as I _________
11. Take the bitter with the _________
12. When one door closes, another one _________
13. You can't judge a book by its _________
14. It's better to give than to _________
15. Good things come in small _________
16. Two heads are better than _________
17. There's no place like _________
18. Don't cry over spilled _________
19. Honesty is the best _________
20. Don't put all your eggs in one _________

Directions: Complete the proverbs. There are at least two words missing.

1. If the shoe fits, _________
2. Time flies when you're _________
3. Don't put off until tomorrow what you _________
4. Absence makes the _________
5. You can't judge a book by _________
6. An apple a day keeps the _________
7. A rolling stone _________
8. The early bird _________
9. No news is _________
10. Don't bite the hand that _________
11. You can kill two birds with _________
12. The best things in life _________
13. People who live in glass houses shouldn't _________
14. A watched pot _________
15. The grass is always greener on the _________
16. A friend in need is a _________
17. Every cloud has _________
18. A little learning is a _________
19. Nothing is certain but _________
20. Cross that bridge when you _________

Directions: Complete the sentence with a word (or words) that makes sense. There are a number of possible answers.

1. Sleep in your ________
2. Take out the ________
3. Climb up the ________
4. Button up your ________
5. Sit in a ________
6. Turn on the ________
7. Knock on the ________
8. Cut with a ________
9. Shave with a ________
10. Fly in a ________
11. Ski down the ________
12. Listen to the ________
13. Plug in the ________
14. Beware of the ________
15. Wade in the ________
16. Clean up your ________
17. Write with a ________
18. Hang up your ________
19. Watch where you ________
20. Load up the ________

Common Phrases

Directions: Complete the phrase with a word (or words) that makes sense. There are a number of possible answers.

1. a bottle of _________
2. a slice of _________
3. a carton of _________
4. a loaf of _________
5. a vase of _________
6. a box of _________
7. a pair of _________
8. a drink of _________
9. a piece of _________
10. an acre of _________
11. a quart of _________
12. a flock of _________
13. a pound of _________
14. a bowl of _________
15. a pot of _________
16. a barrel of _________
17. a glass of _________
18. a nest of _________
19. a group of _________
20. a bar of _________

Directions: Add a word to make a common phrase. There are a number of possible answers.

1. good ________
2. security ________
3. cold ________
4. hand ________
5. national ________
6. double ________
7. sweet ________
8. free ________
9. chocolate ________
10. grand ________
11. talk ________
12. home ________
13. blue ________
14. fire ________
15. high ________
16. first ________
17. French ________
18. sun ________
19. right ________
20. second ________

Word in a Series

Directions: Add a word that would logically follow in the series.

1. morning, noon, _________
2. Tuesday, Wednesday, _________
3. forty, forty-one, _________
4. single, double, _________
5. breakfast, lunch, _________
6. stop, look, _________
7. past, present, _________
8. June, July, _________
9. man, woman, _________
10. 11 o'clock, 12 o'clock, _________
11. penny, nickel, _________
12. zero, one, _________
13. Q, R, _________
14. small, medium, _________
15. breakfast, lunch, _________
16. green light, yellow light, _________
17. autumn, winter, _________
18. beginning, middle, _________
19. sophomore, junior, _________
20. appetizer, salad, _________

Directions: Complete the name of the couple by adding the last name.

1. Romeo and ________
2. Johnny and June Carter ________
3. Lois Lane and Clark ________
4. Bill and Hillary Rodham ________
5. Lucille Ball and Desi ________
6. Prince Charles and ________
7. Fred and Wilma ________
8. Ginger Rogers and Fred ________
9. Mickey and Minnie ________
10. Cinderella and Prince ________
11. Fay Ray and King ________
12. Rhett Butler and Scarlet ________
13. Tarzan and ________
14. Butch Cassidy and the ________
15. Pat Sajek and Vanna ________
16. Miss Piggy and Kermit the ________
17. Adam and ________
18. Snow White and the ________
19. Beauty and the ________
20. George and Laura or George and Barbara ________

Ending Phrases

Expressive: Completions

Directions: Complete the sentence with a word (or words) that makes sense.

1. Lock the door with a ________
2. Wipe your feet on the ________
3. Call a friend on the ________
4. Blow your nose with a ________
5. Dry the dishes with a ________
6. Listen to music on the ________
7. Park the car in the ________
8. Sail the boat on the ________
9. Put a saddle on the ________
10. Buy some food at the ________
11. Set the box on the ________
12. Take the dog for a ________
13. Pour the coffee in the ________
14. Wash your hands with ________
15. Pound the nail with a ________
16. Cook the steak on the ________
17. Sew a button on the ________
18. Spread the butter on the ________
19. Change the tire on the ________
20. Hang the picture on the ________

Directions: Complete the sentence with a word (or words) that makes sense.

1. Eggs are fried in a _________
2. Pictures hang on a _________
3. A letter is mailed in an _________
4. People look at themselves in a _________
5. Bread is cut with a _________
6. Clothes are cleaned in a _________
7. A blanket is put on a _________
8. A bandage is placed on a _________
9. Cake is baked in an _________
10. Money is deposited in a _________
11. Milk is poured from a _________
12. People swim in a _________
13. A printer is hooked up to a _________
14. Bees live in a _________
15. Ice cream is kept in a _________
16. Wine is served in a _________
17. Belts are worn around the _________
18. Cows live in a _________
19. Soup is served in a _________
20. A thermometer tells your _________

Shorter Sentences

Directions: Complete the sentence with a word (or words) that makes sense.

1. The puppy needs to be taken ________
2. Put the ice cream back in the ________
3. Turn left at the ________
4. Most of the tickets were ________
5. She is reading a good ________
6. The sign said *do not* ________
7. I was stung by a ________
8. Would you like a cup of ________
9. The game ended in a ________
10. Target is having a big ________
11. He ripped his new ________
12. He fell asleep on the ________
13. No one laughed at the ________
14. The plumber fixed the ________
15. She prepared a delicious ________
16. His hands were covered with ________
17. The ring had a beautiful ________
18. Weeds were all over the ________
19. My shoulder feels a little ________
20. Wipe the mud off your ________

Directions: Complete the sentence with a word (or words) that makes sense.

1. The robin made a nest in the _________
2. The car stalled in the middle of the _________
3. The lobby has a tank of tropical _________
4. I called the airport to see if the plane will be _________
5. The cat has very sharp _________
6. She has a cold and can't stop _________
7. He ordered grapefruit juice and a bowl of _________
8. Call a plumber to fix the leaky _________
9. The cover story made me want to buy the _________
10. We went to a concert of classical _________
11. The pizza was ordered with onions and _________
12. The baby fell and bumped its _________
13. I swept the dust under the _________
14. She learned to play the piano when she was _________
15. The Red Wings won the hockey game by two _________
16. I sent my sister flowers for her _________
17. John chose a tie to match his _________
18. The vending machine was out of _________
19. The benefit was so successful it raised a million _________
20. Many birds fly south for the _________

General Sentences

Directions: Complete the sentence with a word (or words) that makes sense.

1. The waiter encouraged me to try the ________
2. A small box was delivered to my ________
3. There is a Starbucks just around the ________
4. Someone should go and check on the ________
5. Since no one answered, I left a ________
6. What do you want for your ________
7. The child didn't mean to spill his ________
8. She has a sore throat and a stuffy ________
9. She returned the jacket because it was too ________
10. The soup is pretty bland; it needs some more ________
11. We vacationed in Orlando so the kids could go to ________
12. Although I liked the movie, I thought it was just too ________
13. She searched through her closet looking for a ________
14. They were expecting 60 people at the ________
15. I received a postcard from my ________
16. The water splattered all over the ________
17. I need to pay the bill, but I can't find my ________
18. The concert was rescheduled because the singer was ________
19. There is smoke coming from the ________
20. They are serving baked beans, cole slaw, and grilled ________

Directions: Complete the description with a word that makes sense.

1. The food that bees produce is _________
2. A building where plants are grown is a _________
3. Sixty minutes is one _________
4. The outer part of bread is the _________
5. Seven days make one _________
6. Poker is played using _________
7. The fluid in a pen is called _________
8. Two babies born at the same time are called _________
9. A waiter carries dishes on a _________
10. The loud breathing noise some people make while sleeping is called _________
11. An animal's soft, thick hair is called _________
12. If you think something is funny, it makes you _________
13. Alexander Graham Bell invented the _________
14. Acorns grow on _________
15. Your hand has four fingers and one _________
16. The day after today is _________
17. In a restaurant you choose your food from the _________
18. You stop a car by using the _________
19. Dieting is a way to lose _________
20. Money you earn for doing a job is called _________

Double Phrases

Directions: Think of a word that can follow both words to make a phrase.

1. masking and scotch __________
2. credit and birthday __________
3. sour and whipped __________
4. post and doctor's __________
5. pick-up and garbage __________
6. row and tug __________
7. wedding and boxing __________
8. peer and oil __________
9. tea and surprise __________
10. wind and tread __________
11. cottage and cheddar __________
12. finger and hang __________
13. gold and jelly __________
14. mail and cardboard __________
15. rubber and marching __________
16. permanent and brain __________
17. razor and shoulder __________
18. comic and scrap __________
19. premium and unleaded __________
20. junk and back __________

Double Answers

Directions: Complete the sentence with a word (or words) that makes sense. Then complete the sentence a second time but use another word.

1. Someone left a candy bar on the ________
2. The strong winds blew over the ________
3. The vase held a beautiful bouquet of ________
4. The old dirt road led back to the ________
5. Please cut me a piece of ________
6. There is a long line to get a ________
7. The wall was painted a light ________
8. When it stops raining, we will be able to ________
9. I got a coupon for a free ________
10. My mother and sister are both allergic to ________
11. Tomorrow should be a good day to ________
12. The warehouse got a new shipment of ________
13. Add some chopped garlic to the ________
14. Let me know when you are ________
15. I had a great time at the ________
16. A crowd gathered to look at the ________
17. I have an appointment with my ________
18. He won 60 dollars playing ________
19. She screamed when she saw the ________
20. You get good value for your money at ________

Personal Thoughts

Directions: Complete the sentence so it applies to you.

1. Before I get too old, I would like to . . .
2. After saving my family in a fire, I would save . . .
3. Two people from history I would like to talk with are . . .
4. The place I have enjoyed living most is . . .
5. If I had the opportunity and the ability to change careers, I would become . . .
6. For a special treat I would like to . . .
7. If I could change one of my habits, I would change . . .
8. If I won a week's all-expenses-paid trip to any state, I would go to . . .
9. What I like most about myself is . . .
10. Most people don't know I am really very . . .
11. The most stressful time of my life was when . . .
12. On weekends, my favorite method of relaxation is . . .
13. I would like more natural ability in the area of . . .
14. As a child, my favorite toy or book was . . .
15. If my life were made into a movie, I would have me played by . . .
16. Most people don't know that I can . . .
17. Aside from good health near the end of my life, I would like to have . . .
18. If I had judicial power, I would require tougher sentences for . . .
19. If I could redo one room in my home, it would be . . .
20. You can tell when I'm upset because . . .

Directions: Complete the sentence with several words.

1. It was too early to . . .
2. She waved at . . .
3. They had lunch before they . . .
4. It was not legal to . . .
5. Don't leave until . . .
6. The package was delivered . . .
7. It was the worst . . .
8. Even though they were married, . . .
9. Let's walk to . . .
10. The salesperson guaranteed that . . .
11. It was hard to choose between . . .
12. When was the last time you . . .
13. The rumor is that . . .
14. Who wants to . . .
15. He asked for the manager because . . .
16. It won't be long before . . .
17. She believed the president when . . .
18. I want to thank everyone for . . .
19. After he finished painting, . . .
20. He doesn't eat lobster because . . .

Directions: Complete the sentence with a word (or words) that makes sense.

1. Anticipate a _________
2. Eliminate the _________
3. Criticize the _________
4. Strain the _________
5. React to the _________
6. Experiment with the _________
7. Contradict the _________
8. Intercept the _________
9. Register the _________
10. Decorate the _________
11. Blame it on the _________
12. Honor the _________
13. Diagnose the _________
14. Flatten the _________
15. Inspire the _________
16. Refuse the _________
17. Complain to the _________
18. Witness the _________
19. Transfer the _________
20. Organize the _________

NAMING

Directions: Answer the questions.

1. What city do you live in?
2. What is your address?
3. How tall are you?
4. What is your shoe size?
5. What color are your eyes?
6. What are your parents' first names?
7. What was the last school you attended?
8. What was your mother's maiden name?
9. What city and state were you born in?
10. When is your birthday?
11. What is your telephone number?
12. What bank do you use?
13. Name a medication you take.
14. Name any brothers or sisters you have.
15. What is your primary doctor's name?
16. What is the name of your health insurance company?
17. What was your father's occupation?
18. (if applicable) What are your children's and / or grandchildren's names?
19. (if applicable) What is your spouse's name? Name his or her family members.
20. (if applicable) What kind of pet(s) do you have? What are the names?

Basic Words in Common

Directions: Add a word that fits with the other words.

1. cardinal finch _________
2. nephew cousin _________
3. soccer ball bowling ball _________
4. June September _________
5. poodle retriever _________
6. lasagna pizza _________
7. trout cod _________
8. windy cloudy _________
9. triangle square _________
10. Smith Johnson _________
11. sidestroke breaststroke _________
12. pint gallon _________
13. Labor Day Fourth of July _________
14. Dr. Pepper 7-Up _________
15. chin nose _________
16. Reagan Kennedy _________
17. Spain Italy _________
18. spider centipede _________
19. Coast Guard Air Force _________
20. gall bladder kidney _________

Directions: Name a word that fits with the other words.

1. Emmy Grammy Tony _________
2. track court rink _________
3. *Gourmet* *Cosmopolitan* *Newsweek* _________
4. lieutenant colonel ensign _________
5. turkey sweet potatoes cranberry sauce _________
6. torch lantern flares _________
7. shrimp cocktail stuffed mushrooms cheese ball _________
8. blender coffeemaker Crock-Pot _________
9. Sears Penney's Macy's _________
10. Taurus Cancer Leo _________
11. Lady Bird Johnson Dolly Madison Betty Ford _________
12. *All My Children* *As the World Turns* *General Hospital* _________
13. twine ribbon wire _________
14. orangutan rhesus chimp _________
15. blackjack keno roulette _________
16. Motrin Advil Excedrin _________
17. cancer diabetes lupus _________
18. Visa Discover American Express _________
19. king queen twin _________
20. clipping offsides double fault _________

Directions: Think of one word that can be placed after each of the three words to make new words.

1. speeding, parking, admission _________
2. electric, folding, high _________
3. moth, volley, eye _________
4. cheese, devil's food, coffee _________
5. barbed wire, chain link, picket _________
6. address, comic, check _________
7. paper, doggie, garment _________
8. main, Sesame, one-way _________
9. law, three-piece, bathing _________
10. egg, Caesar, potato _________
11. button, pot, cubby _________
12. apple, tomato, tartar _________
13. court, bird, green _________
14. baking, curry, talcum _________
15. face, fork, weight _________
16. Hawaiian, night, long-sleeved _________
17. sales, income, property _________
18. candle, chop, drum _________
19. animal, oyster, nut _________
20. paddle, spinning, steering _________

Directions: Name a category into which all three words fit.

1. root beer ginger ale club soda
2. gray green gold
3. ring bracelet pin
4. pig cow chicken
5. sapphire emerald ruby
6. clarinet trumpet saxophone
7. Houston St. Louis Omaha
8. pistachio almond cashew
9. Stanford Harvard Princeton
10. crayons markers pencils
11. Ford Cadillac Toyota
12. wool corduroy cotton
13. egg roll fried rice fortune cookie
14. leopard elephant gorilla
15. wrench pliers hammer
16. sandals sneakers moccasins
17. whole wheat pita rye
18. garlic cinnamon basil
19. impatiens marigolds geraniums
20. mop vacuum dust rag

Name the Category

Directions: Name a category into which all three words fit. Be specific.

1. split pea soup guacamole lime jello
2. World Cup Wimbledon The Masters
3. Bit-O-Honey Oh Henry! PayDay
4. hotel dormitory nursing home
5. shuffleboard croquet horseshoes
6. weddings slicing onions sad movies
7. piano keys penguins Oreo cookies
8. triathlon relay race marathons
9. root canal filling bridge
10. nitrogen helium carbon monoxide
11. ostrich flamingo stork
12. rabbit's foot the number 7 4-leaf clover
13. ladybugs dice dalmatians
14. mousse gel conditioner
15. malpractice personal injury tax
16. key chains T-shirts postcards
17. porthole sunroof skylight
18. snakes heights spiders
19. Lifesavers M & Ms jellybeans
20. fax copier computer

Directions: Watch me as I demonstrate each item. Then tell me what I am doing.

1. playing a piano
2. waking up and stretching
3. standing up
4. taking a shower
5. drinking a beverage
6. putting on boots
7. blowing my nose
8. coughing
9. brushing my teeth
10. hammering a nail
11. hitting a golf ball
12. rowing a boat
13. diving into a pool
14. fixing a tie
15. eating something that is too hot
16. horseback riding
17. conducting an orchestra
18. jogging in place
19. sneezing
20. walking up stairs

Basic Antonyms

Directions: Name a word with the opposite meaning.

1. beginning
2. lost
3. worst
4. false
5. shallow
6. warm
7. early
8. ladies
9. enter
10. noisy
11. win
12. first
13. clear
14. high
15. morning
16. light
17. crooked
18. weak
19. rich
20. empty

Directions: Name a word with a similar meaning.

1. intelligent
2. large
3. highway
4. sob
5. begin
6. inexpensive
7. soiled
8. assist
9. champion
10. mad
11. lady
12. ill
13. overweight
14. pal
15. simple
16. pretty
17. physician
18. amusing
19. glad
20. weak

Antonyms

Directions: Name a word with the opposite meaning.

1. defense
2. cause
3. appreciative
4. artificial
5. accept
6. vertical
7. skeptic
8. pain
9. spend
10. reward
11. clumsy
12. permanent
13. complain
14. gradually
15. listen
16. contemporary
17. cheerful
18. boring
19. flabby
20. conclusion

Directions: Name a word with a similar meaning.

1. annoy
2. demolish
3. prohibit
4. essential
5. furious
6. ethical
7. consent
8. broad
9. precisely
10. impartial
11. shatter
12. peculiar
13. melody
14. reluctant
15. concluded
16. anxious
17. remedy
18. brook
19. wager
20. instruct

Product Brands

Directions: Name a product or type of product associated with the brand name.

1. ExxonMobil
2. Tide
3. FedEx
4. Hoover
5. Verizon
6. Dannon
7. American Express
8. Jockey
9. ebay.com
10. Rogaine
11. Gillette
12. Nabisco
13. Duracell
14. Kenmore
15. Michelin
16. Olympus
17. Hershey
18. Special K
19. Hummer
20. Charmin

Directions: Name a product associated with the name.

1. George Foreman
2. Ralph Lauren
3. Oscar Meyer
4. Ben & Jerry
5. Dr. Scholl
6. Harley Davidson
7. Mrs. Fields
8. Jenny Craig
9. Eddie Bauer
10. Benjamin Moore
11. Jack Daniels
12. Orville Redenbacher
13. Mrs. Butterworth
14. Denny's
15. Black & Decker
16. Ethan Allen
17. Betty Crocker
18. Mrs. Dash
19. Barnes & Noble
20. Swiss Miss

Directions: Answer the questions.

What would you use to . . .

1. weigh yourself
2. help you see better
3. fuel a car
4. cool a drink
5. light a fire
6. clean your hair
7. protect a cut
8. rest your head on
9. brush your teeth
10. cool a room
11. blow your nose
12. dry your hands
13. clean dirt off a floor
14. lock a door
15. get to the tenth floor of a building
16. keep your hands warm
17. make an omelet
18. water a garden
19. fix your hair
20. see in the dark

Directions: Name something that the items are associated with.

What you think of when you hear . . .

1. caller ID and voice mail
2. home plate and pitcher's mound
3. shells and sand
4. drive-thru window and French fries
5. molars and dentures
6. gingerbread house and candy canes
7. jokers and aces
8. mast and rudder
9. bifocals and contact lens
10. bib and high chair
11. commercials and reruns
12. handlebars and pedals
13. windshield wipers and speedometer
14. lizards and cacti
15. lipstick and mascara
16. jury box and witness stand
17. wishbone and drumsticks
18. AM and FM
19. Eiffel Tower and Notre Dame
20. beard and mustache

Functions

Directions: Answer the questions.

What is used to . . .

1. help make objects and print look bigger?
2. store leftovers in a freezer?
3. cut grass?
4. help the police catch speeding motorists?
5. help you move the cursor around a computer screen?
6. make a cord reach an outlet?
7. pick up hot dishes?
8. make a wood surface smooth?
9. model clothes in a store window?
10. make a room or a house less dry?
11. hit a croquet ball?
12. wipe spilled liquid from a table?
13. cover up unpleasant odors in a room?
14. wrap a sprained ankle / wrist?
15. play Yahtzee or Backgammon?
16. cut through the skin in surgery?
17. check the oil level in a car?
18. walk a dog in public?
19. make antipasto?
20. clean between each tooth?

Directions: Explain where or why these words would be written.

1. Two months' security deposit required
2. 50¢ daily / $2.00 Sunday
3. Add $5 for shipping and handling
4. 200 calories per 6 oz. serving
5. Manufacturer's suggested retail price
6. No exchange without receipt
7. No wake
8. Adults only
9. Do not sell after July 2009
10. Do not remove under penalty of law
11. Valid ID required
12. Warranty expires at 60,000 miles or 5 years
13. Par 3
14. Handicapped parking
15. Loading zone
16. This side up
17. Emergency Entrance
18. Baggage Claim
19. Exact change required
20. This is a paid political announcement

Word Clues

Directions: Name something that the three words taken together suggest.

1. defendant, jury, decision
2. harness, rip cord, free fall
3. face, hair, lips
4. mercury, fever, Fahrenheit
5. gargle, rinse, fresh breath
6. salty, snack, twisted
7. Triple Crown, race, Lexington
8. product, scented, armpit
9. Ellis Island, torch, France
10. babies, disposable, smelly
11. teens, dating, clock
12. feet, clippers, ingrown
13. storm, wind, twister
14. jacket, penguin, rent
15. boat, motion, nauseous
16. breakfast, links, meat
17. February, shadow, Punxsutawney
18. bear, black and white, China
19. fuzzy, larva, butterfly
20. hops, on tap, alcohol

Directions: After the first clue, name a word that could fit the description. Add the first clue to the second one and name a word that would fit both clues. Combine the third clue along with the first two and name a word that fits with all three clues.

1. It is a part of your body. It is in your mouth. It contains the taste buds.
2. These are eating utensils. They are often made of wood. They originated in China.
3. It is an earth-shattering event. It is of great concern in California. It occurs along a fault line.
4. It is a snack food. It comes in a small box. The box also contains a small prize.
5. It is an animal. It is about the size of a groundhog. It shoots its quills when it is attacked.
6. It is protective equipment. It is worn by construction workers. It is worn on the head.
7. You do it with your hands. You do it when pleased. You do it after a good performance.
8. It is found in the ocean. It is a legendary creature. It is half-woman, half-fish.
9. It is a type of fruit. It has a hard shell. It is grown on palm trees.
10. It is a mark on the skin. It can be small or large. It is the result of the skin being cut.
11. It has your picture on it. It has to be renewed. You need it to travel between countries.
12. It is a dairy product. It comes in a carton. It can be creamed, small curd, or large curd.
13. It is a type of boat. It goes back and forth between two points. It carries cars as well as people.
14. It is a type of reptile with scales. Its bite is poisonous. It makes a noise by vibrating its tail.
15. It is women's clothing. It is worn in the water. It has two skimpy pieces.
16. It is a sound made by a person. It can be soft or loud. It is done when asleep.
17. It is a plant or small shrub. You would not want it in your garden. It can give you a rash if you touch or rub against it.
18. Two people do it. It is done instead of having a marriage ceremony. A justice of the peace is usually involved.
19. It is an unpleasant condition. It is generally associated with aging. It is caused by inflammation and pain in the joints.
20. They are entertainers. They perform in front of people. They make people laugh.

Attractions

Directions: Name a place in the United States that is suggested by the clues.

1. the city with cable cars and the Golden Gate Bridge
2. the name of a national park in the Rockies with Old Faithful
3. the city known for car production and Motown music
4. the natural attraction at the New York–Canadian border that people have tried to go over in barrels and other strange things
5. the city known for gambling and lavish hotels on the Strip
6. the home of Elvis Presley in Memphis that millions tour through
7. the city that hosts Mardi Gras and has the French Quarter
8. the huge rock formation and park where people can hike or take mules down to its base
9. the address of the home of the president of the United States
10. the place in New York City from which the countdown to the new year takes place
11. the city with the Freedom Trail and Harvard
12. the peninsula of Massachusetts that is an especially popular place in summer
13. the city with the Sears Tower and the home of the Bulls and the Bears
14. the large park in the middle of New York City
15. the largest city in the island state
16. the national educational institution in Washington D.C. that includes 18 museums
17. the Pennsylvania city known for having cheesesteaks and the Liberty Bell
18. the place in Massachusetts where the Pilgrims landed in 1620
19. the city with the Grand Ole Opry and the Country Music Hall of Fame
20. the place in Florida where space shuttles are launched from

Directions: Answer the questions with the name of a well-known person.

Who is or was . . .

1. the creator of Mickey Mouse and his theme park
2. a French artist who cut off his own ear
3. the current host of *The Tonight Show*
4. a president associated with freeing the slaves after the Civil War
5. an entertainer who hosted an annual Labor Day Telethon for many years
6. the woman who is an expert at cooking, crafts, and anything involved with homemaking
7. the dictator of Cuba often pictured with a cigar in his mouth
8. the wealthiest man in America and the founder of Microsoft Company
9. the president who was impeached, resigned, and pardoned after the Watergate scandal
10. the mayor of New York City during the terrorist attack in 2001
11. the female talk-show host who once gave a new car to each person in her audience
12. an Italian artist who painted the Sistine Chapel
13. a wealthy New Yorker known for his real-estate dealings and as host of *The Apprentice*
14. a past president from Texas whose son was also president
15. the person who made the Model T and whose car company still carries his name
16. the woman who hosted *The Today Show* before she took an evening news anchor position
17. the man who invented electricity and the record player at his Menlo Park laboratory
18. the Saudi Arabian head of the Al Qaeda terrorist organization
19. the former general and chairman of the Joint Chiefs of Staff who was secretary of state during the New York City terrorist attack
20. the legendary singer, actor, and director who will always be known for the song *People* and her portrayal of Fanny Brice in *Funny Girl*

Well-Known Names

Directions: Name someone who fits the description.

1. an older singing group that still performs
2. the name of a song with a person's name in it
3. a movie star over the age of 45
4. a very wealthy family
5. a famous person with a beard
6. a famous bald person
7. a movie with an animal's name in the title
8. a celebrity who appears on TV ads
9. a singing duo
10. a senator's name
11. a fairy-tale character
12. an actor (male or female) who dances well
13. a deceased artist whose paintings are now worth millions
14. a character from a Shakespearean play
15. a famous person who died young
16. someone who goes by one name
17. someone who goes by three names—first, middle, and last
18. a new remake of a previously released movie
19. two names that are probable presidential nominees of either party
20. a celebrity known more for physical appearance than for his or her acting

Directions: Answer the question.

1. What is the fluid pumped by the heart?
2. What needs to be tied on some shoes?
3. What are white flakes on the scalp called?
4. What is a topping for ice cream?
5. What is the capital of the United States?
6. What is a coin worth 25¢?
7. What is used to stick things on metal?
8. What is the coldest season of the year?
9. What is used to look up the meaning of a word?
10. What is a nickname for William?
11. What holiday is celebrated in September?
12. What is an eight-legged insect that spins a web?
13. What is a period of 100 years called?
14. What is put around property to keep people from trespassing?
15. What animal looks for his shadow on February 2?
16. What swings back and forth on a grandfather clock?
17. What do you look at to see your reflection?
18. What are you supposed to find at the end of the rainbow?
19. What follows lightning?
20. What is used to repair a hem?

Basic Definitions

Directions: Name a word that fits the description.

1. put off until later
2. give money or goods to a cause
3. a sandy shore
4. talk very softly
5. your name written in script
6. come back into view
7. a partner in crime
8. things to be thrown out
9. a small, green Irish elf
10. a group of guiding principles
11. take into custody
12. what blood travels through
13. say you are sorry
14. a gem found in oysters
15. set in one's ways
16. no feeling in a part of the body
17. cook in hot oil
18. the backbone
19. a sound caused by indigestion
20. items in a recipe

Directions: Name a word that fits the description.

1. a tool needed to open a bottle of wine
2. the division between two states or countries
3. a very dark shade of red
4. tiny beads of water that run off the skin
5. a bone that is cracked but not broken
6. an Italian soup with lots of vegetables
7. the state of being in a trance but still able to take suggestions
8. material made from the hide of a cow
9. chosen out of the blue, in no particular order
10. the message on a triangular traffic sign meaning to give the right of way
11. what horses' feet are called
12. an item put in reading material so that a page can be found
13. pieces of material that fall from space and land on Earth
14. a classic board game using letter tiles to form words on a board
15. the organ in the body that filters oxygen when we breathe
16. to stop something from happening
17. the front part of a theater where the concessions are
18. what it is called when a man asks a woman to marry him
19. flowers that come up each year
20. the part of a printed page left blank on either side and at the top and bottom

Definitions 2

Directions: Name a word that fits the description.

1. a type of sale in which the person who offers the most money gets the item
2. an hour-by-hour plan for a trip, tour, or seminar
3. the term for when an innocent person is held captive by someone
4. the official notice of a person's death
5. the name given to horns on deer, elk, and moose
6. tedious jobs that need to be done daily
7. the lever on a gun that is pulled back in order to fire it
8. a decoration etched on the body using a needle and ink
9. what some people can play on others, especially on April 1
10. advertisements that interrupt TV or radio shows
11. the place where beer is made
12. money received when an item is returned
13. a painting or drawing of someone's face
14. a term for someone who says one thing but then does something else
15. an item used to serve from a punch bowl
16. a small line used to divide some written words
17. small brownish dots on someone's face or body
18. money that is earned from an investment
19. liquid produced by the mouth that we continually swallow
20. to see or hear something that has no basis in reality

Directions: Answer the questions.

1. What do you call the foam produced from soap and water?
2. What do you call the two long, pointed teeth on either side of the front teeth?
3. What material makes tape stick?
4. What is an eating disorder that results in people becoming too thin?
5. What is the term for a person who travels the same long route to and from work?
6. What is it called when people dissolve their marriage legally?
7. What is the process called when water turns into steam and disappears?
8. What is the small tool used to pluck out unwanted hairs or splinters?
9. What are the names of two pieces on a chessboard?
10. What do you call a small, round replica of the earth?
11. What term describes a house inhabited by ghosts?
12. What is the lower part of your chin in which your teeth are embedded?
13. What kitchen appliance can dice, chop, or mash food?
14. What do you call the tiny fish that are sometimes added to pizza?
15. What is the communication called that uses the hands to form letters and words?
16. What is the sound a wolf makes at the moon?
17. What are the parts called that you separate in a garlic bulb?
18. What is the material called that is put in walls and ceilings to help save energy costs?
19. When something comes out of the clothes dryer smaller than when it went in, what happened to it?
20. What is the middle joint in the finger called?

Descriptions 1

Directions: Name a word that fits the description.

1. a shelf above a fireplace
2. your father's sister to you
3. surface imprints left by people or animals
4. a stretchy material used in the waistbands of some pants
5. a method of helping someone who has stopped breathing
6. an award of money given to a student to help pay for college
7. a technique to relieve pain using long, thin needles that are inserted into the skin
8. a condition as a result of a blow to the head
9. the word that defines a golf score that is one under par
10. an intriguing story usually about a person that is passed among several people
11. the term for a person who has more than one spouse
12. what a check-out clerk scans on a product
13. someone who cannot read or write
14. a book written by an author about the author's life
15. the official opening of a movie, usually with the stars present
16. grilled pieces of meat or vegetables on a skewer
17. the general type of drugs taken to help get rid of an infection
18. a party given for a bride before her wedding
19. the ingredient that gives guacamole its green color
20. money that is passed off as authentic but is not

Directions: Answer the questions.

1. What is a person with a negative outlook called?
2. What does *expecting* mean when referring to a woman?
3. What is an exact copy of something called?
4. What word means to try out for a part in a production?
5. What is the job title for someone hired to keep another person safe from harm?
6. What do you call a sudden outburst of temper?
7. What word describes something very easily broken?
8. What is someone called who can do things with either hand?
9. What is a term for a young child who knows more than expected at that age?
10. What exercise is between walking and running in speed?
11. What is the substance inside a bone called?
12. What is the condition when a person does not remember his or her past?
13. What are people exposed to who are near others using cigars or cigarettes?
14. What is the word for a viewpoint often considered cautious, traditional, or old-fashioned?
15. What is the term for a fairly good guess of an amount?
16. What does a small *c* in a circle on a page mean?
17. What type of food poisoning can you get from raw or undercooked food from animals?
18. What is a group of people singing together called?
19. What is the term for money you pay to take a class?
20. What type of puzzle has many interlocking pieces?

Descriptions 3

Directions: Name a word that fits the description.

1. This car gauge tells how fast you are going.
2. This is applied to dry or flaky parts of the body to soften them.
3. This system is installed in some offices and public places so people can communicate throughout an area or listen to music.
4. These are worn on the pupil of the eye to help someone see better.
5. This is the first formal class in school that a child attends.
6. This part of a horse's harness is held to control the animal's movements.
7. This is used to sweeten drinks without adding calories.
8. This is used in stores to ring up sales and hold money and change.
9. This is added to a load of wash to whiten or brighten clothes.
10. This is worn over clothing especially while cooking to protect against spills.
11. This is used on lawns to keep them healthy.
12. This cheese is often grated over spaghetti and pasta dishes.
13. This procedure is done to fingernails or toenails to make them look better.
14. These are used to stick notes on refrigerators.
15. This is the noise a dog makes when it is upset.
16. This device will warn you if there is a fire in your home.
17. This is a nonstick finish used on many cookware items.
18. This is the final practice before a performance.
19. This is the surface on which ice hockey is played.
20. This piece of paper proves graduation from a school.

Directions: Name one word that fits both definitions.

1. to gulp **and** a small bird
2. a place to swim **and** a game using a cue stick
3. a flap on men's pants **and** a buzzing insect
4. a dried fruit **and** to trim a tree or bush
5. a female name **and** to bring a legal case against
6. a playing card **and** a garden tool
7. to make a knot **and** to finish at the same time
8. an herb **and** a place where money is made
9. the skin of an animal **and** to put out of sight
10. a group of words **and** a punishment
11. loud noises **and** tennis equipment
12. a type of tree **and** a part of the hand
13. a type of meat **and** a show-off
14. not dangerous **and** a place to keep valuables
15. a vegetable **and** to crush
16. to cut nails **and** to fasten together
17. to fill a suitcase **and** a group of wolves
18. a small storage building **and** to be rid of hair
19. a recreational area **and** to leave a car
20. a container **and** to fight

Dictionary Defined

Directions: *Name a word that fits the definition. The information in brackets gives the first letter of the answer and what part of speech it is. The bracketed information could be used only if needed.*

1. Wash or clean by rubbing hard. [S, verb]
2. An area of deep water protected from wind and current by barriers and that forms a safe place for ships to anchor. [H, noun]
3. Distinctive clothes worn by the members of a group when on duty. [U, noun]
4. To conduct oneself in a specified way; to act well. [B, verb]
5. Anything that is burned to give heat or power. [F, noun]
6. A series of musical tones that form a tune. [M, noun]
7. Tangy liquid produced by the fermentation of cider or wine. [V, noun]
8. To injure the ligaments or muscles of a joint by a sudden twist or wrench. [S, verb]
9. To start a fight with; strike out at someone. [A, verb]
10. To own up to one's sins; to admit one's guilt. [C, verb]
11. To make drawings or marks absentmindedly while talking or thinking. [D, verb]
12. Something thrust into a person's mouth to keep him from talking or crying out. [G, noun]
13. To choose for an office by voting. [E, verb]
14. A person who is on the other side in a fight, game, or discussion. [O, noun]
15. A kind of shoe made of a sole fastened to the foot by straps. [S, noun]
16. The part of the body between the ribs and the hips. [W, noun]
17. Paste-like mixture that hardens when dry and is used for covering walls and ceilings. [P, noun]
18. Easy to read; plain and clear writing. [L, adjective]
19. Capable of being turned inside out; made so that either side can be used. [R, adjective]
20. A broad roadway lined with trees; a wide street or thoroughfare. [A, noun]

WORD FLUENCY

Directions: Name some things in the category. The first category is a basic one. The words in brackets can be added to the category to define it even more.

1. animals [with short tails]
2. colors [pastels]
3. fruit [with a pit]
4. body parts [that can be transplanted]
5. clothing [with zippers]
6. movies [musicals]
7. medications [that are prescription-only]
8. tools [for garden and yard work]
9. sports [that use a net]
10. jobs [where most of the work involves standing]
11. countries [in Europe]
12. insects [without wings]
13. flowers [that come in several colors]
14. games [played on a board]
15. transportation [without wheels]
16. beverages [that are served chilled]
17. things in a kitchen [that plug in]
18. actors [who are deceased]
19. breakfast foods [eaten hot]
20. musical instruments [that you blow into]

Foods

Directions: Name several foods that fit the description.

1. cookies
2. cereals
3. pasta and noodle dishes
4. toppings for burgers
5. soups
6. salad ingredients
7. cheeses
8. nuts
9. pizza toppings
10. three-course meals
11. main dishes
12. sandwiches
13. foods you eat without utensils
14. snack foods
15. ice cream flavors
16. vegetables you cook and don't eat raw
17. syrups and sauces
18. foods with eggs as an ingredient
19. foods to put garlic and / or onions in
20. one dish from each ethnic variety you can think of

Directions: Name several parts to each item listed.

Name several parts of . . .

1. your face
2. newspaper
3. engine
4. theater
5. airplane
6. hospital
7. your insides (internal organs)
8. refrigerator
9. orchestra
10. salad bar
11. car
12. house
13. fireplace
14. library
15. set of dishes
16. toolbox or a sewing kit
17. horse
18. grocery store or supermarket
19. elementary school
20. stove

Basic Supplies

Directions: Name some of the equipment or supplies you need to complete the task.

Name things you need to . . .

1. do laundry
2. make a salad
3. wrap a gift
4. play a pick-up game of baseball
5. furnish a living room
6. protect yourself from the sun's rays
7. decorate a holiday tree or have a child's birthday party
8. start a vegetable garden
9. prepare your tax returns
10. make a banana split
11. set a table
12. organize your stuff
13. care for a canary or a parakeet
14. go on a picnic
15. play a round of golf
16. make spaghetti
17. build a bonfire
18. make a quilt or a bookcase
19. clean a bathroom
20. paint a room

Directions: Name some equipment, characteristics, and duties associated with the jobs.

Name things you associate with . . .

1. artists
2. mechanics
3. police officers
4. surgeons
5. soldiers
6. priests
7. accountants
8. actors
9. dentists
10. reporters
11. pharmacists
12. lifeguards
13. veterinarians
14. magicians
15. attorneys
16. nurses
17. senators
18. teachers
19. carpenters
20. store owners

Directions: Name some television shows from the past or present that fit the description.

1. prime time shows
2. shows in which you learn how to do something
3. shows with the main character's name in the title
4. TV families we got to know from the show
5. shows that are televised once a year
6. cable channels
7. reality shows
8. shows that stayed on many years
9. game shows
10. shows from the 50s and 60s
11. shows that are on Thursday night
12. sports shows scheduled at least weekly
13. shows featuring detectives or lawyers
14. cartoon or animated TV shows
15. shows televised at 10:00 P.M. or later
16. soap operas
17. shows that are on five days a week
18. PBS shows
19. people who started on TV shows and became famous
20. cast members or characters from *Saturday Night Live*

Directions: Name some brand names that belong with the product.

1. shoes
2. laundry detergents
3. moisturizing lotions
4. dog or cat food
5. underwear
6. butter or margarine
7. washers and dryers
8. beer or wine
9. household cleaning products
10. over-the-counter pain relievers
11. shampoo
12. televisions
13. bottled water
14. paper products
15. men's clothing
16. jewelry
17. frozen dinners
18. watches
19. cheese
20. spaghetti sauce

Companies

Directions: Name several companies that fit the description.

1. computer and computer-related companies
2. phone companies
3. soft drink companies
4. pizza companies
5. car companies
6. nonprofit organizations
7. furniture companies
8. home-building companies
9. companies that do business over the Internet
10. insurance companies
11. airline companies
12. mortgage companies
13. drug companies
14. companies that went bankrupt or were bought out
15. candy and chocolate companies
16. cosmetic companies
17. investment companies
18. real estate companies
19. publishing companies
20. overnight delivery companies

Directions: Name some ingredients that are used to make each food.

1. tossed salad
2. stew
3. omelet
4. stuffing or dressing for a turkey
5. meat loaf
6. minestrone
7. granola
8. birthday cake
9. spaghetti sauce
10. potato salad
11. Greek salad
12. Reuben sandwich
13. apple crisp
14. hot fudge sundae
15. lasagna
16. barbecue sauce
17. cheesecake
18. New England clam chowder
19. chili
20. homemade cookies (you choose the kind)

Visualizing

Directions: Name some things that you associate with each place. It might help to visualize being in the setting and name what you visualize around you.

1. forest
2. carnival or state fair
3. Disney's Magic Kingdom
4. bowling alley
5. courtroom
6. fitness club
7. Comerica Park or other large stadium
8. airport terminal
9. cathedral or other religious institution
10. bakery
11. post office
12. cafeteria
13. zoo
14. dentist's office
15. building construction site
16. McDonald's, Wendy's, or Burger King
17. the Las Vegas strip
18. TV studio taping a live show
19. inside a mall
20. flea market

Directions: Name some things associated with each item.

Name things you associate with . . .

1. a new baby
2. a jungle
3. retirement
4. rock bands
5. the music industry
6. poverty
7. cruise ships
8. Paris
9. computers
10. 1600 Pennsylvania Avenue, Washington, D.C.
11. casinos
12. graduation
13. wealth or luxury
14. Hollywood
15. the Red Cross
16. politicians
17. airplanes
18. a major holiday (pick one)
19. Iraq
20. teenagers

Locations

Directions: Give some specific names of places in the United States that fit the description.

1. national parks
2. colleges and universities
3. mountains
4. restaurant chains
5. famous buildings
6. vacation spots
7. largest cities by population
8. smallest states by size
9. theme parks or family entertainments spots
10. cities on an ocean
11. hotel and motel chains
12. places associated with music, singers, or concerts
13. places to see in California
14. places to see in New York City
15. places to see in Florida
16. places to see in Washington D.C.
17. largest American companies
18. stores that are nationwide chains
19. locations where movies or TV shows have taken place
20. natural and man-made landmarks

Directions: Name some places where you might see the items.

Name places where you could . . .

1. see vending machines
2. enter only if you are a member
3. see rows of seats
4. see long lines
5. get together with friends
6. view special exhibits
7. see more men than women
8. see many cars
9. rest and relax
10. find antiques
11. see groups of children
12. hear music performed
13. buy or sample lots of different foods at one place
14. see security guards
15. have a wedding reception
16. see trash
17. find dust and cobwebs
18. see people in uniforms
19. go fishing
20. buy items at a low price

Well-Known People

Directions: Name some people (past or present) who fit the description.

1. professional athletes
2. film directors
3. artists
4. singers
5. fashion designers
6. comedians
7. inventors
8. composers
9. religious leaders of different faiths
10. good-looking celebrities
11. people who have run for a state or national position and lost
12. actors who have won a lot of awards
13. romantic lead actors (male and female)
14. actors whose movies require a lot of stunts and are action-packed
15. people who have written bestsellers
16. older musicians who are still touring
17. retired athletes who have other jobs
18. people who are or were known as part of a team such as Johnny Carson and Ed McMahon
19. people who give advice to others via TV, radio, or books
20. people who are known for supporting a particular cause

Directions: Name some items that fit the description.

1. things to pack on a trip to a lake or ocean
2. things to pack on a skiing trip
3. things to pack to go camping
4. things to pack for a cruise
5. things to pack when traveling with an infant
6. things to pack when going to Wisconsin in January
7. things to pack when going to Phoenix in July
8. things to take for an outdoor evening concert on the grass
9. things to pack for a cross-country car trip
10. thing to pack when flying to stay with an old friend for a week
11. things to pack in an overnight bag
12. things to store in an attic
13. things to keep in a toiletry kit or cosmetic bag
14. things to carry in a gym bag
15. things to carry in a purse or business case
16. things that should be kept in your car
17. things you should always have with you when you travel
18. things to have in a first-aid kit
19. things to have ready at home in case the power goes out
20. things to keep in a safe

Personal Information 1

Directions: Name some items that fit the description.

1. things you sometimes get a craving for
2. things you do more on weekends than on weekdays
3. things that make you nervous
4. little things people do that annoy you
5. things you do when you want to relax
6. things you would like to own but would not buy
7. items you have but seldom use
8. things you never have the time to do
9. places where you shop or eat fairly often
10. clothing you have but rarely wear
11. things that tire you out or things that energize you
12. foods you eat too much of
13. things you leave out on your counters (bathroom, kitchen, dresser)
14. things you like about the area in which you live
15. places you have no interest in visiting
16. things that were popular when you were growing up that are not popular now
17. phrases you use a lot
18. classes you have taken and enjoyed
19. sounds you like listening to
20. things you find boring to do or watch

Directions: Name some items that fit the description.

1. things you have that you don't ever want to part with
2. things you wanted to do when you were young but have no desire to do now
3. valuable lessons you learned growing up
4. words you would use to describe your mother
5. things you would do if you had the money, resources, or time
6. good qualities you feel you have
7. things you are grateful for
8. things you didn't do or learn growing up that now you wish you had
9. favorite places you went to as a child
10. friends you had while you were growing up
11. people you enjoy being with
12. toys you enjoyed playing with as a child
13. teachers who made an impact on you
14. events in your life that have shaped who you are today
15. people in the news who have had an influence on you
16. good memories you have from high school
17. things you remember about your old neighborhood(s)
18. what you and your siblings or you and your parents argued about
19. questions you would like to ask your parents but probably won't
20. people you knew in your life who had the most influence on you

Mixed Categories 1

Directions: Name some items that fit the description.

1. ways people waste time
2. facial expressions
3. celebrities who you don't believe deserve their fame
4. significant events in American history
5. important inventions and products of the twentieth century
6. people whose jobs it is to help you look your best
7. medications you do not swallow
8. causes for which people raise money
9. issues about which men and women often disagree
10. shows or acts associated with Las Vegas
11. methods of sending information to another person
12. symbols associated with holidays
13. fillings in a box of chocolates
14. famous or infamous crimes
15. celebrity couples who have broken up or are no longer married
16. three-letter living things
17. events at which you take photographs
18. love songs
19. ways to use duct tape
20. phrases that are overused

Directions: Name some items that fit the description.

1. things that make you blink
2. things you buy in pairs
3. things people put on walls besides pictures
4. things you need two or more people in order to do
5. things you need to replenish or replace on a regular basis
6. things that are hard to find if they are dropped
7. things a doctor checks or orders during a physical exam
8. things used to hold other things
9. things that will hurt if you touch them
10. things that should be done while wearing protective gloves
11. things that run on batteries
12. things that come in powdered form
13. things you recycle
14. things you can do to increase the value of your house
15. things people do while they are driving
16. things people use once and don't use again
17. things you need to use a key to open besides doors
18. things that make your heart beat fast
19. things that make you laugh
20. things that need your signature in order to be valid

Naming by Action

Directions: Name some items that fit the description.

Name things you can . . .

1. slice
2. file
3. polish
4. stuff
5. roll
6. catch
7. peel
8. write
9. melt
10. spray
11. plant
12. burn
13. read
14. paint
15. climb
16. pour
17. staple
18. fry
19. dissolve
20. inflate

Directions: Name some items that fit the description.

Name things that have . . .

1. claws
2. pockets
3. handles
4. springs
5. shells
6. wrinkles
7. holes
8. covers
9. feathers
10. seats
11. roots
12. stripes
13. expiration dates
14. horns
15. beards
16. signs
17. blades
18. photos in them
19. initials on them
20. numbers on them

Naming by Modifier

Directions: Name some items that fit the description.

Name things that are . . .

1. sticky
2. hard to hold
3. kept frozen
4. fuzzy
5. sharp
6. adjustable
7. dangerous
8. smoked
9. hard to understand
10. bought by the pound
11. awarded to people
12. often stolen
13. habit-forming
14. carved
15. flat
16. tossed
17. delivered to your door
18. elastic
19. transparent
20. handed down to the next generation

Directions: Name some items that fit the description.

1. stores where you would never shop
2. magazines you do not read
3. movies you have no interest in watching
4. fashions or clothing you would never wear
5. things that do not grow naturally in your area
6. things you would not do if you wanted to relax
7. places you would not want to live
8. foods you do not like
9. things to do if you cannot fall asleep
10. people you would not trust
11. sports you do not enjoy watching
12. chores you have never liked doing
13. places where you would not go because you would feel uncomfortable
14. things that are not polite to do
15. things you do not like about the area in which you live
16. things men do not like to talk about
17. things women do not like to admit
18. jobs you would not like to do for a living
19. celebrities you do not have any interest in hearing about
20. traits you would not want your children to have

Directions: Name some items that fit the description.

1. things you appreciate more as you get older
2. things you put up with rather than do something to change
3. things people worry about even though worrying won't do any good
4. things cats would do that dogs would not
5. things you can do at night better than during the day
6. things that are easier to do in water than out of water
7. things that are easier to understand if you watch rather than read about them
8. things that are different colors on the outside than on the inside
9. things a child can do that adults have trouble doing
10. things that look the same upside down as they do right-side up
11. things that appear to be more complicated than they are
12. things you wouldn't do but wish you had the nerve to do
13. things that would hurt if you touched them
14. things you can recognize by their smell
15. things that look better in the dark than in daylight
16. things that are too tall for short people
17. things you do in your own home that you would not do in someone else's
18. things you never have been able to do that you wish you could do
19. things that women can do that men cannot do
20. things that look better the more you see of them

Directions: Name some reasons that might cause the item to occur.

Name reasons to . . .

1. call the police
2. go to a hospital
3. be arrested
4. move to a new location
5. go on a diet
6. change jobs
7. start exercising
8. go on the Internet
9. get rid of some of your possessions
10. do volunteer work
11. take a trip
12. stand in line
13. take pills
14. have a party
15. lie down
16. turn off the TV
17. carry a cell phone
18. get a pet
19. be on a waiting list
20. rent rather than buy

Philosophical Questions

Directions: Name some items that fit the description.

1. good values to teach a child
2. problems facing America today
3. things people take for granted in life
4. traits that help people cope with life's tougher times
5. events from the past that helped shape the future of America
6. valuable things that you cannot buy
7. things older people like to reminisce about
8. lessons teenagers sometimes learn the hard way
9. things we do today that your great-grandparents would never have thought possible
10. well-known people who are good role models
11. things parents should do for their children
12. things children should do for their parents
13. ways to be a good neighbor
14. qualities of a good mother
15. qualities of a good father
16. qualities of a good teacher
17. qualities of a good boss or supervisor
18. qualities of a good leader
19. qualities you look for in a mate
20. qualities you look for in a friend

Directions: Name some words that have nearly the same meaning as the one given.

1. humorous
2. underweight
3. miserable
4. strange
5. elated
6. administrator
7. wages
8. dirty
9. additional
10. money
11. pliable
12. chuckle
13. love
14. intelligence
15. massive
16. approximately
17. slow
18. attractive
19. alike
20. communicate

Directions: Name some words that fit the description. An example or two is shown in parentheses.

1. two-word cities (Des Moines)
2. words beginning with *BR* (broken)
3. compound words (drawbridge)
4. words whose plural does not just add an *s* (box—boxes, ox—oxen)
5. repeatable four-letter words (golly)
6. fruits and vegetables that begin with *P* (parsnips)
7. two-word phrases *(all clear, no exit)*
8. words that begin and end with the same letter (Oreo, river)
9. words that have double letters (bottle, boot)
10. letters of the alphabet that are also words (Q = cue)
11. states beginning or ending with a vowel (West Virginia)
12. one-word movie or TV titles (*Titanic, Friends*)
13. word pairs but not opposites (brush and comb)
14. rhyming words or phrases (cookbook, super duper)
15. people whose first and last names start with the same letter (Ronald Reagan)
16. people who use initials in their names (T. S. Eliot)
17. words that rhyme with straight (great)
18. three-letter words starting with D (dry)
19. words that can follow the word *over* (overalls)
20. words or phrases that include colors (the Golden Rule)

SENTENCE FORMULATION

Directions: Make a sentence using all three words.

1. buy, car, Monday
2. lived, farm, Illinois
3. ate, muffin, breakfast
4. wash, plate, sink
5. reserve, tickets, play
6. watch, movie, Friday
7. locked, keys, car
8. this, bag, mine
9. please, coffee, cream
10. get, aspirin, drugstore
11. mother-in-law, called, visit
12. hotel, weekend, north
13. new, book, lost
14. closet, paint, bedroom
15. hope, weather, hot
16. write, letter, company
17. fell, broke, ankle
18. dig, worms, fish
19. meet, friend, tomorrow
20. hamburger, fries, lunch

Directions: Make a sentence that includes the word.

1. bruises
2. limit
3. trailer
4. hike
5. secret
6. lake
7. garlic
8. hug
9. memory
10. field
11. employees
12. sunburn
13. plot
14. speakers
15. puzzle
16. jokes
17. germs
18. rocks
19. option
20. catnap

Directions: Make a sentence that includes all the words.

1. apples, healthy, dessert, serve
2. announce, half, liquidate, sale
3. discovered, rare, disease, research
4. robber, teller, note, money
5. children, measles, scratch, scars
6. sauce, beef, butter, boil
7. bulbs, Holland, bury, order
8. Williamsburg, colonial, tourist, blacksmith
9. cousin, wrote, visit, month
10. trophy, football, first, season
11. locked, neighbor, lost, home
12. spiders, fear, web, legs
13. rose, petals, dry, bouquet
14. nursery, child, licensed, five
15. briefcase, papers, seminar, Tuesday
16. crop, citrus, frost, Texas
17. subscription, news, expire, renew
18. leather, bag, imported, cost
19. vase, glass, fell, pieces
20. reruns, rent, movie, TV

Directions: Make a sentence that includes some form of the verb.

1. ignore
2. pass
3. pretend
4. crush
5. shuffle
6. apologize
7. frustrate
8. repair
9. create
10. deny
11. forget
12. understand
13. scrub
14. remove
15. give out
16. analyze
17. promise
18. handle
19. admire
20. prevent

Directions: The start of a sentence is given. Complete the sentences with more words.

1. What was the . . .
2. Don't forget to . . .
3. The guide explained the . . .
4. There weren't any . . .
5. Tell me when you . . .
6. I tried to . . .
7. Give me the . . .
8. The weather predicted . . .
9. The men have . . .
10. I don't believe . . .
11. One of these days . . .
12. I hope you . . .
13. Sometimes it is . . .
14. Have you been . . .
15. Public servants are . . .
16. You can get . . .
17. The mosquito bit . . .
18. It is supposed to . . .
19. We won't be . . .
20. Which one does . . .

Directions: Make a sentence that includes each phrase.

1. during the show
2. without getting tired
3. for good luck
4. before the storm
5. along the edge
6. next to the
7. is pretty good
8. not without my
9. when he said
10. in spite of
11. across the street
12. lots of water
13. under the table
14. with a sharp knife
15. in the mail
16. with my mother
17. for an hour
18. at the airport
19. on a diet
20. by the way

Directions: Make a sentence that includes each phrase.

1. small print
2. a change of pace
3. car pool
4. up to date
5. department store
6. out of order
7. parking meters
8. maximum security
9. upside down
10. soccer practice
11. federal government
12. left-handed
13. spoiled rotten
14. book review
15. voice mail
16. false alarm
17. keep tabs on
18. odds and ends
19. get the nerve
20. run-down buildings

Mixed Words

Directions: Make a sentence that includes the word.

1. convinced
2. squeaky
3. damp
4. suburbs
5. regular
6. profitable
7. imagination
8. nervous
9. miracle
10. valuable
11. scrambled
12. complicated
13. twisted
14. fancy
15. military
16. trouble
17. dizzy
18. flexible
19. impossible
20. secret

Directions: Make one sentence that includes both of the words.

1. mail, male
2. hair, hare
3. write, right
4. board, bored
5. week, weak
6. won, one
7. waist, waste
8. steel, steal
9. cents, sense
10. chews, choose
11. blew, blue
12. close, clothes
13. rose, rows
14. would, wood
15. guessed, guest
16. heal, heel
17. wee, we
18. through, threw
19. pairs, pears
20. knows, nose

Conditional Words

Directions: Make a sentence that includes the word.

1. absolutely
2. maybe
3. without
4. except
5. almost
6. because
7. might
8. only
9. between
10. neither
11. rattling
12. supposed to
13. as long as
14. weird
15. especially
16. through
17. yet
18. next to
19. beyond
20. less

Directions: Explain about each item.

1. What is a calendar?
2. What is a rainbow?
3. What is a sweatshirt?
4. What are Post-It-Notes?
5. What is a scab?
6. What are gutters?
7. What is a statue?
8. What is a refund?
9. What is canvas?
10. What is a recipe?
11. What are knuckles?
12. What is a mortgage?
13. What is a shredder?
14. What is a patio?
15. What is a pulse?
16. What are floor plans?
17. What is dandruff?
18. What is a search warrant?
19. What are cosmetics?
20. What is a subway?

Name a Use

Directions: Explain what each item is used for.

1. shutters
2. tent
3. shower cap
4. bookends
5. ACE bandage
6. coupons
7. steel wool
8. blueprint
9. toothpicks
10. dry ice
11. fireplace screen
12. aluminum foil
13. placemats
14. sawhorse
15. caulk
16. shingles
17. debit cards
18. inner tubes
19. skylight
20. Saran Wrap

Directions: Explain what you associate with each item.

1. Sesame Street
2. Pentagon
3. French Quarter
4. Franklin Mint
5. Williamsburg
6. Supreme Court
7. Salvation Army
8. Wall Street
9. Times Square
10. Eiffel Tower
11. Super Bowl
12. Afghanistan
13. National Enquirer
14. Amazon.com
15. Hurricane Katrina
16. Academy Awards
17. Vatican
18. Carnegie Hall
19. Mayo Clinic
20. Boston Tea Party

Relationships

Directions: Explain the relationship between the two people and why they are linked together.

1. Clark Kent and Superman
2. Henry Ford and the Model T
3. Dr. Seuss and the Cat in the Hat
4. Tarzan and Jane
5. Rush Limbaugh and Howard Stern
6. Batman and Robin
7. Lewis and Clark
8. Dorothy and Toto
9. James Bond and 007
10. Bambi and Thumper
11. Adam and Eve
12. Charlie Brown and Snoopy
13. Ben and Jerry
14. Bill Clinton and Al Gore
15. Gepetto and Pinocchio
16. Barbie and Ken
17. Scarlett O'Hara and Rhett Butler
18. Humpty Dumpty and Little Miss Muffet
19. Maria and the Von Trapp family
20. Cookie Monster and Big Bird

Directions: Explain what the television show is about. Pick one of the two shows listed in each question.

1. *Meet the Press* or *Face the Nation*
2. *All in the Family* or *I Love Lucy*
3. *Antiques Roadshow* or *This Old House*
4. *Survivor* or *American Idol*
5. *Entertainment Tonight* or *Access Hollywood*
6. *Queer Eye for the Straight Guy* or *Larry King Live*
7. *M*A*S*H* or *Cheers*
8. *Cosby* or *All in the Family*
9. *Hardball* or *The O'Reilly Factor*
10. *Emeril Live* or *Iron Chef*
11. *Jeopardy* or *Wheel of Fortune*
12. *America's Funniest Home Videos* or *Extreme Makeover: Home Edition*
13. *Law & Order* or *CSI: Crime Scene Investigation*
14. *The Simpsons* or *The Flintstones*
15. *Lost* or *24*
16. *Oprah* or *Ellen*
17. *Friends* or *Everybody Loves Raymond*
18. *America's Most Wanted* or *Cops*
19. *Primetime* or *Dateline NBC*
20. *ER* or *Grey's Anatomy*

Define Words

Directions: Explain about each item.

1. What is a caterer?
2. What are steroids?
3. What is a mutual fund?
4. What is acne?
5. What is a corridor?
6. What is arthritis?
7. What is sushi?
8. What are flip-flops?
9. What is charisma?
10. What is a defibrillator?
11. What does sarcastic mean?
12. What does trivial mean?
13. What does soothing mean?
14. What does sentimental mean?
15. What does exotic mean?
16. What does allegedly mean?
17. What does spontaneous mean?
18. What does creative mean?
19. What does impulsive mean?
20. What does organic mean?

Directions: Explain the meaning and why the item is important.

1. Heimlich maneuver
2. Velcro
3. franchise
4. daylight savings time
5. plagiarism
6. Alaskan Pipeline
7. acupuncture
8. advanced directives
9. endangered species
10. alimony
11. West Nile virus
12. OnStar
13. Dove bars
14. lottery
15. power of attorney
16. bariatric surgery (gastric bypass)
17. Taser weapons
18. smoothies
19. Google
20. statute of limitations

Cause for a Comment

Directions: Explain the circumstances that might cause someone to make the statement.

1. It must be a slow news day.
2. That squirrel might have rabies.
3. It must have rained during the night.
4. I need a smaller size.
5. Don't go near the windows.
6. Citizen's arrest.
7. I think I am going to faint.
8. Excuse me, but I was next.
9. It's not a good day to go sailing.
10. I can't believe this is happening to me.
11. This shirt should be washed right away.
12. It's amazing. You haven't changed a bit after all these years.
13. I'm sure that's not a real diamond.
14. I wish I had practiced more.
15. Ouch! Cut it out.
16. That must be a special order.
17. This is not a safe neighborhood.
18. Hold your breath.
19. You are never satisfied.
20. Yes, dear.

Directions: Explain what the sentence means in your own words.

1. He got up on the wrong side of the bed.
2. You are the spitting image of your mother.
3. His channel surfing drives me crazy.
4. I can read you like a book.
5. Let's call it a day and go to happy hour.
6. I have to work the graveyard shift next week.
7. After three days of snow, I have a bad case of cabin fever.
8. The old refrigerator finally bit the dust.
9. The name of the movie is on the tip of my tongue.
10. He got cold feet the week before his wedding.
11. Many of my friends are empty-nesters.
12. My uncle is a real couch potato.
13. I've felt down in the dumps all week.
14. John wishes he could get rid of his beer belly.
15. I'm going to catch 40 winks before the party.
16. That piece of apple pie really hit the spot.
17. Keep your fingers crossed that I'll get the job.
18. We're having trouble making ends meet.
19. The bottom line is that the design doesn't have a chance of winning.
20. The reporter had an off-the-record conversation with the judge.

Directions: The answer is given. Tell what the question might be and under what circumstances it would be said.

1. Not in this lifetime.
2. Ten percent.
3. 48 to 36—the Lakers trail the Pistons.
4. Weekdays 9 to 6. Saturday 10 to 5. Closed Sundays.
5. Ranch, please, but on the side.
6. 140 over 75.
7. We sold the last one an hour ago.
8. Cloudy with a 30 percent chance of rain.
9. Area code 313-555-1234.
10. A tall decaf hazelnut latte.
11. Twenty-eight days except in leap year.
12. Just a little bit to the left.
13. Closing at 28, down 2¼.
14. Medium rare.
15. A 60 watt and a 100 watt.
16. 1.2 karats in white gold.
17. By midnight at the latest.
18. Stop worrying.
19. I have it totally under control.
20. I take the Fifth.

Directions: Answer the question in a full sentence.

1. When do you get a new mattress?
2. When do most people retire?
3. When do you take a nap?
4. When do most people write a will?
5. When would you call an exterminator?
6. When is a good time to buy a new car?
7. When does someone get a bachelor party?
8. When would a metal detector be used?
9. When would you have a tree taken down?
10. When is a good time to buy stock?
11. When would you have lots of leftovers?
12. When would you file an insurance claim?
13. When do you go through customs?
14. When do you need bifocals?
15. When would you donate blood?
16. When would you need a notary public?
17. When can someone begin to collect Social Security?
18. When do you take your temperature?
19. When do you save a receipt?
20. When would you respond to a survey?

Why Questions

Directions: Answer the question in a full sentence.

1. Why do people take supplements?
2. Why would you buy a carbon monoxide detector for your whole home?
3. Why are more communities allowing legalized gambling (casinos)?
4. Why do we have a federal income tax?
5. Why do some foods need to be refrigerated?
6. Why do many offices have fax machines?
7. Why do insurances have different deductible rates?
8. Why do some criminals get several life sentences?
9. Why do people use lotion on their skin?
10. Why does Las Vegas have so many wedding chapels?
11. Why do people get flu shots?
12. Why do some people count calories?
13. Why do some people have their cats declawed?
14. Why do we have real estate agents?
15. Why do we have discount outlets?
16. Why do states have lotteries?
17. Why do we use carbon monoxide detectors?
18. Why do many places have drive-thru windows?
19. Why do people dye their hair?
20. Why are many TV shows on for one season or less?

Directions: Answer the question by giving at least one example.

1. When would you use a copy rather than an original?
2. When would you accept a meal at a restaurant rather than send it back?
3. When would you borrow something rather than buy it?
4. When would you hire a professional rather than do the job yourself?
5. When would you pay in cash rather than charge it?
6. When would you pay a traffic ticket rather than fight it?
7. When would you take a train or bus rather than drive yourself?
8. When would you postpone rather than go to an interview?
9. When would you go in person rather than call?
10. When would you pay for tickets rather than accept free ones?
11. When would you see a doctor rather than treat yourself?
12. When would you screen your calls rather than answer your telephone?
13. When would you have your house cleaned rather than clean it yourself?
14. When would you elope rather than have a wedding?
15. When would you get carryout rather than make a meal?
16. When would you drive to the hospital rather than dial for emergency help?
17. When would you walk in a group rather than alone?
18. When would you buy something for full price rather than shop for a discount?
19. When would you donate a piece of furniture rather than resell it?
20. When would you rent a house rather than buy it?

Directions: Answer the question in a full sentence (or sentences).

What would you say . . .

1. to get a waiter's attention
2. to a mugger who wants your money
3. to a lost and crying child
4. when returning a damaged product to a store
5. to someone you caught lying to you
6. to someone you are attracted to
7. to someone you bumped into by mistake
8. when meeting a movie star
9. to someone you don't want to see again
10. after someone gives you a gift
11. if you were told you won a lot of money
12. when apologizing for a misunderstanding
13. to someone who complimented you on your outfit
14. to a police officer who stops you
15. to a store clerk who gives you the wrong change
16. to someone turning 100 years old
17. to someone at your door asking you to sign a petition
18. to the president of the United States
19. to someone who is going to cut your hair
20. to a rude salesclerk who was having a personal phone conversation while you were trying to get information and buy something

Directions: Answer the question with your reasons.

1. Do you like to travel by air? Why or why not?
2. Do you like big gatherings of people? Why or why not?
3. Do you like new technology and electronic gadgets? Why or why not?
4. Do you like to work on craft projects? Why or why not?
5. Do you like to go sailing? Why or why not?
6. Do you like to eat breakfast? Why or why not?
7. Do you like to sing in the shower? Why or why not?
8. Do you like to try new recipes or foods? Why or why not?
9. Do you like to travel and see new places? Why or why not?
10. Do you like to play solitaire? Why or why not?
11. Do you like to follow a pro sports team? Why or why not?
12. Do you like to follow celebrity gossip? Why or why not?
13. Do you like to gamble or go to casinos? Why or why not?
14. Do you like to exercise? Why or why not?
15. Do you like to collect things? Why or why not? If so, what do you collect?
16. Do you like everything in order with no clutter? Why or why not?
17. Do you like reading autobiographies? Why or why not?
18. Do you like science fiction and thinking about the future? Why or why not?
19. Do you like going to live concerts? Why or why not?
20. Do you like the state of the world today? Why or why not?

Past Facts

Directions: Answer the question with details.

1. What was your first paying job? Explain how you got it and what you did.
2. What was the neighborhood like where you grew up?
3. What is the first birthday party that you remember?
4. What do you remember about the elementary school you attended?
5. When you were growing up, what was your favorite thing to eat?
6. Who gave you your first kiss?
7. If you had pets, which one was your favorite?
8. What article of clothing do you remember hating to wear?
9. What was your best family vacation while you were growing up?
10. What was the first car you remember your family having?
11. Who was your favorite relative and why?
12. If you had a brother or sister, what did you tease him or her about (or vice versa)?
13. When did you get your best grades in school?
14. Who was your favorite teacher and why?
15. What was your favorite subject in high school and why?
16. Who was your first big crush?
17. What was a nickname you had and how did you get it?
18. What was your favorite toy and what happened to it?
19. What were your high school colors and team name?
20. Who was your best friend growing up and what did you like to do?

Directions: Answer the question with your opinion and why you feel that way.

What do you think is . . .

1. the best chocolate treat and why
2. the worst recent meal you have had that you paid for and why
3. the best brand of ice cream and why
4. the worst country to live in and why
5. the best two TV shows you have seen and why
6. the worst month of the year and why
7. the best pizza and why
8. the worst teacher you ever had and why
9. the best ride at an amusement park and why
10. the worst food for you that you enjoy the most and why
11. the best singing group and why
12. the worst event in history and why
13. the best product that makes some chore easier and why
14. the worst job for you that you could have and why
15. the best cities in which to live and why
16. the worst trip you ever took and why
17. the best cure for the hiccups and why
18. the worst regret you have in your life and why
19. the best advice you ever got and why
20. the worst fear you have and why

Directions: Decide which answer is a better fit for you and explain why.

1. Which interests you more—history or science?
2. Which is more difficult for you—writing a speech or giving a speech?
3. Which do you like better—Italian or Chinese food?
4. Which do you think is more desirable—health or wealth?
5. Which involves more of your time—preparing yearly taxes or paying monthly bills?
6. Which is faster for you—adding on paper or using a calculator?
7. Which do you prefer for sleeping—open windows or air conditioning?
8. Which do you prefer—working with computers or working with people?
9. Which is easier for you to do—draw or sing?
10. Which do you prefer taking—a shower or a bath?
11. Which do you prefer—feeling too hot or too cold?
12. Which do you prefer listening to—AM or FM radio?
13. Which would you rather do—hold political office or manage a small company?
14. Which would you prefer to play—the lottery or slot machines?
15. Which do you think is a more desirable pet—a dog or a cat?
16. Which climate do you like better—Florida or Arizona?
17. Which extra room would you prefer having—a home gym or a screened-in porch?
18. Which would be harder for you to give up—listening to the radio or watching TV?
19. Which is harder for you to control—your appetite or your temper?
20. Which would you prefer—a great body or a great mind?

Directions: The first sentence sets up the situation. ***Assume that is true*** *and answer the question based on the situation.*

1. You complain about a neighbor. What are you upset about?
2. You are packing for a vacation. When and where are you going?
3. You are called to the principal's office. What did you do?
4. A foundation is started in your honor. What cause will it help?
5. You are moving out of state. Why and where?
6. You decide to take up a hobby. What is it and why did you choose it?
7. You have a black eye. What happened?
8. You take part in a rally. What are you protesting?
9. You get mad at a child. What did the child do?
10. You apologize to your wife or husband. What did you do?
11. You don't have your wallet with you. Where did you leave it?
12. You get tickets to a concert. Who is performing and where?
13. You throw out food that has gone bad in your refrigerator. What are you throwing out?
14. You finally make that commitment you have been putting off for a long time. What is the situation and why have you been putting it off?
15. You receive a summons to appear in court. Why?
16. You ask someone to stop doing one thing that annoys you. What is it and why is it annoying?
17. You make contact with someone you have not seen for a long time. Who is it and why did you choose this person?
18. You are really motivated to change one habit. What is the habit and why do you want to change it?
19. You request a very special breakfast. What will you be having?
20. You are getting new living room furniture. Why?

LONGER ANSWERS

Directions: Use the word in at least two sentences with two completely different meanings.

1. set
2. mold
3. bat
4. rock
5. well
6. falls
7. shed
8. track
9. dated
10. fair
11. second
12. strike
13. leaves
14. block
15. ring
16. fly
17. straw
18. trunk
19. slip
20. kind

Make a Story

Directions: Make up a story that has the items listed in it. Tell the story and make sure all of the words are included at least once. [Give up to four words or add more words of your own].

1. rabbit, diamond ring, lantern, joke
2. half-hour, dumpster, knees, official
3. advice, period, crystal, dome
4. khaki, aching back, signs, license
5. surface, machine, bankrupt, cheddar
6. thunderstorm, manners, Iowa, rehearsal
7. cough drops, personality, box office, questions
8. floor, dolphins, ivory, oranges
9. ice, post office, exercise, rotten
10. rivals, emergency room, briefcase, paid
11. regrets, dates, stand, defective
12. digested, jar, flirt, necessary
13. kicked, affair, national, independent
14. balancing, elbows, peppermint, lucky
15. dedicated, silence, sale, French
16. refused, survival, guests, permanent
17. crush, innocent, reward, better
18. depend, mask, miniature, adjustable
19. incompatible, jeans, weeds, elastic
20. organize, profitable, identical, original

Directions: Choose something in the category named, but don't say the word you are thinking of. Give clues to describe the item until I guess your word.

1. color
2. wild animal
3. sport
4. dessert
5. article of clothing
6. type of jewelry
7. appliance
8. bird
9. TV show
10. state
11. vegetable
12. actor
13. piece of furniture
14. musical instrument
15. body part
16. country
17. beverage
18. farm animal
19. holiday
20. flower

Visual Descriptions

Directions: Describe the item in detail without saying any words from its name. I will guess based on your description. Describe it as if you were talking to someone who is blind.

1. lizard
2. scarecrow
3. sand castle
4. skunk
5. crutches
6. turtleneck sweater
7. traditional wedding cake
8. palm tree
9. kangaroo
10. grand piano
11. peacock
12. snail
13. Eiffel Tower
14. toaster
15. hockey puck
16. basset hound
17. Mona Lisa
18. harp
19. banana split
20. octopus

Directions: Choose an answer and explain your choice, including your reasons why. Include a reason why you don't like the other choice.

Would you rather . . .

1. see a movie or a stage play
2. have a pedicure or a facial
3. eat steak or salmon
4. live in a warm climate or in one with changing seasons
5. go to a restaurant or prepare your own meal
6. travel across country by train or by car
7. play a board game or a card game
8. go to bed early and get up early or go to bed late and get up late
9. lose your sight or your hearing
10. watch a comedy or a drama
11. watch a sport or play the sport
12. go out on a Friday night or stay home and relax
13. live in a new home or an old but remodeled home
14. be musical or artistic
15. see a movie in the theater or rent it and watch it at home
16. live in a city or in the country
17. have a flexible schedule and go into work or do your work from home
18. do the laundry or vacuum
19. watch a football or a basketball game
20. live in a slow-paced or fast-paced area

Directions: Choose the activity you think is more difficult and give at least two reasons why.

Which is harder . . .

1. being a good parent or being a good spouse
2. cleaning a fish or cleaning a turkey
3. spending time with someone who likes to talk or someone who likes to listen
4. lifting weights or jogging
5. raising a boy or raising a girl
6. accepting a compliment or accepting a favor
7. growing flowers or vegetables
8. living in an unhappy marriage or getting a divorce
9. cross-country skiing or downhill skiing
10. playing *Jeopardy!* or playing *Wheel of Fortune*
11. writing a speech or giving a speech
12. spending time with an eight-year-old or time with a teenager
13. memorizing a poem or memorizing a joke
14. painting a room or wallpapering a room
15. planning and shopping for a meal or preparing a meal
16. cutting sugar or cutting fat from your diet
17. writing a sympathy note or writing a thank-you note
18. getting rid of things you no longer use or organizing the things you have
19. dusting or vacuuming
20. gaining weight or losing weight

Directions: Put the items in order from what you think is least to most desirable and give reasons for why you ranked each item as you did.

1. In what order would you enjoy winning:
   money a trip furniture
2. In what order would you enjoy a weekend getaway to:
   a cottage on a lake a hotel in New York City camping in a national park
3. In what order would you like tickets to a:
   zoo theme park museum
4. In what order would you like a vacation in:
   Philadelphia St. Louis Seattle
5. In what order would you like a letter from:
   the IRS wedding invitation a friend
6. In what order would you like a subscription to:
   People *Time* *Reader's Digest*
7. In what order would you take up as a hobby:
   furniture refinishing playing an instrument scrapbooking
8. In what order would you volunteer time in:
   an animal shelter a nursing home a library
9. In what order would you support:
   Cancer Society AIDS research Heart Association
10. In what order would you be interested in buying:
    pick-up truck luxury car SUV
11. In what order would you enjoy watching:
    documentary game show comedy
12. In what order would you enjoy an evening out for:
    dinner at a nice restaurant drinks with friends bowling
13. In what order would you enjoy living in:
    a large city a college town a small community
14. In what order would you wish to have:
    a great disposition a great intellect a great sense of humor
15. In what order would you enjoy:
    reading walking watching TV

16. If you had the money, in what order would you invest in:
    antiques stock real estate

17. In what order would you prefer eating:
    sushi Thai food Indian food

18. In what order would you want to have dinner with:
    Oprah Winfrey George Clooney Bill Clinton

19. In what order would you enjoy season tickets to professional:
    hockey basketball football

20. In what order would you have these surgeries:
    hip replacement liposuction a root canal

Directions: Identify who would be likely to make the statement and explain under what circumstances it would be said.

1. Checkout time is noon.
2. Gentlemen, start your engines.
3. When I was a child, I had to walk barefoot five miles uphill to school.
4. May I see your driver's license and a major credit card?
5. You have the right to remain silent, the right to have an attorney . . .
6. Three windows and installation will run you about $1,400.
7. Everyone must stay behind the barricade.
8. I see a long life ahead of you filled with great wealth.
9. The specials of the day are meat loaf and roast chicken.
10. The call-in number to vote for your favorite is . . .
11. We have Bud, Michelob, and Miller on tap.
12. It's a girl.
13. Press 2 if you have questions about your account.
14. What is the last thing you remember before the accident?
15. N–34.
16. The seat belt sign has been turned off in the main cabin.
17. Our top story tonight is . . .
18. Play ball.
19. Sign here on the dotted line.
20. Do you provide health insurance or other benefits?

Figures of Speech 1

Directions: Explain what each phrase means and give an example of how you would use each phrase.

1. yard sale
2. fair-weather friend
3. sweet tooth
4. red tape
5. penny pincher
6. open house
7. bridal shower
8. tourist trap
9. first lady
10. pack rat
11. backseat driver
12. catnap
13. car pool
14. fender bender
15. green thumb
16. rain check
17. junk mail
18. blind date
19. nest egg
20. poker face

Directions: Explain the meaning of the phrase in your own words, then give an example of when it would be used in real life.

1. Save it for a rainy day.
2. Better late than never.
3. It's easier said than done.
4. It was love at first sight.
5. Money is no object.
6. Read between the lines.
7. The squeaky wheel gets the grease.
8. That's the last straw.
9. Keep a stiff upper lip.
10. Don't rock the boat.
11. Get off my back.
12. Let bygones be bygones.
13. Keep your fingers crossed.
14. Go off the deep end.
15. Take it or leave it.
16. It's water over the dam.
17. You get what you pay for.
18. No man is an island.
19. Take the bull by the horns.
20. Give it your best shot.

Directions: Answer the question with at least two different details about the person.

Who are these people?

1. Tiger Woods
2. Bill Gates
3. Colin Powell
4. Paul McCartney
5. John McCain
6. Michael Jordan
7. Rolling Stones
8. George Walker Bush
9. Meryl Streep
10. Aretha Franklin
11. Faith Hill and Tim McGraw
12. Al Gore
13. John Travolta
14. Condaleeza Rice
15. Ron Howard
16. Tom Hanks
17. Martin Luther King, Jr.
18. Rosie O'Donnell
19. Rachel Ray
20. Barack Obama

Directions: Explain how each item is used and give an example of when or why it is used.

1. casters
2. dehumidifier
3. treadmill
4. blood transfusion
5. suction cups
6. cell phone
7. coasters
8. motion detector lights
9. hassock or ottoman
10. medical alert systems (bracelets or emergency response systems)
11. citronella candles
12. invisible fence
13. halogen bulbs
14. grout
15. phone card
16. solar panels
17. shredder
18. awnings
19. dry ice
20. trellis

Directions: Use full sentences to give the following information about the place: where it is, what you associate with it, why it is important, and what it looks like (as appropriate).

1. the Alamo
2. Ellis Island
3. Old Faithful
4. Graceland
5. Air Force One
6. Betty Ford Clinic
7. Kennedy Space Center at Cape Canaveral
8. Rose Bowl
9. EPCOT Center
10. Arlington National Cemetery
11. Empire State Building
12. Playboy Mansion
13. the Mint at Fort Knox
14. Panama Canal
15. Martha's Vineyard
16. Amish areas of the country
17. World Trade Center
18. the Mall of America
19. Capital Building
20. Martha's Vineyard or Nantucket

Directions: Explain how each item is used and give an example of when or why it is used.

1. frequent flyer miles
2. ethanol
3. fax machine
4. hybrid cars
5. Home Shopping Network
6. Post-It Notes
7. Viagra
8. cellulite
9. call waiting
10. MP3 Player
11. digital camcorders
12. Prozac
13. WebCam
14. Bluetooth headsets
15. flat-panel HDTV
16. Rogaine
17. airbags
18. CAT scan
19. Botox injections
20. roll-ups or wrap sandwiches

Directions: Use full sentences to give the following information about the item: what it is, what you associate with it, why it is important, and any controversies associated with it.

1. stem cell research
2. wireless technology
3. hybrid cars
4. terrorism
5. death penalty
6. United Nations
7. paparazzi
8. Supreme Court
9. Homeland Security
10. border patrols
11. National Guard
12. social security
13. cloning
14. identity theft
15. global warming
16. domestic violence
17. West Nile virus or Avian (bird) flu
18. Internet predators
19. Patriot Act
20. public schools and education

Directions: Listen to the situation and answer the questions.

1. *You are in a post office to buy a roll of stamps.*
   What would the clerk say?
   What would you say?

2. *You are in a hospital bed and a nurse comes over to you.*
   What would the nurse say?
   What would you say?

3. *You are cashing a check in a bank.*
   What would the teller say?
   What would you say?

4. *You have just witnessed a hit-and-run car accident.*
   What would you say to a police officer?
   What would the officer say to you?

5. *You are trapped in an elevator with two strangers.*
   What would you say?
   What would you not want either of them to say?

6. *You approach a counter where someone is offering free food samples.*
   What would you say?
   What would the person say?

7. *You are seated in a restaurant's nonsmoking section and a person next to you lights up a cigar.*
   What would you say?
   What would the person probably say?

8. *You are introduced to your state senator.*
   What would the senator say?
   What would you say?

9. *You are singing along to the radio and your spouse walks in the room.*
   What would your spouse say?
   What would you say?

10. *You sit down at a bar.*
    What would the bartender say?
    What would you say?

11. *You are at a professional baseball game and sitting next to a spectator who catches a foul ball.*
    What would the person who caught the ball say?
    What would you say?

12. *You have not paid your car payment and receive a letter from the finance company.*
    What would the letter say?
    How would you respond?

13. *A young child asks you how he was born.*
    What would you say?
    What would the child probably respond?

14. *You are paying your bill in a nice restaurant when you learn your credit card has been declined.*
    What would the clerk say?
    What would you say?

15. *You help a disabled person cross the street.*
    What would the person say?
    What would you say?

16. *You open your door to a Federal Express courier with a large envelope.*
    What would the courier say?
    What would you say?

17. *You are out of gas in a boat on a big lake and another boater yells to see if you need help.*
    What would you say?
    What would the boater say?

18. *You give an envelope to the bride and groom at their reception.*
    What would you say?
    What would they say?

19. *You are having bad back pain and call a specialist who your friend likes.*
    What would you say to the receptionist?
    What would the receptionist say?

20. *You think you want to learn to golf.*
    What would you say to a pro before having a first lesson?
    What would the pro say?

Directions: Answer the question in full sentences. Think of at least three questions you would ask for each situation.

What questions would you ask . . .

1. before you buy a used car
2. before donating to a cause
3. if you are comparing phone companies
4. if you are applying for a part-time job
5. if you are buying a puppy
6. before you sign a petition
7. before you join a fitness club
8. before you vote for a candidate
9. before you hire a person to do work around your home
10. before you join a bowling league
11. before you go to a newly released movie
12. before you hire a decorator to remodel a room in your home
13. before you enroll your child in a daycare center
14. before you book and pay for plane tickets
15. before you go on a first date
16. a pharmacist about a new medication you will be taking
17. before you buy season tickets to a professional sports team
18. before you make reservations at vacation resort
19. when you meet new neighbors
20. when you are deciding between models of refrigerator

Reverse Descriptions

Directions: Give me information about the topic without saying its name so that I will be able to understand what you are talking about. Include specific details as requested, and follow the other instructions.

1. Describe a TV show by its story line.
2. Describe a tourist attraction but don't say its name or exactly where it is.
3. Describe a movie star only by giving the names of characters he or she has played.
4. Describe a fairy tale but don't say its title.
5. Describe something in your refrigerator without saying its name.
6. Describe a female you know by her mannerisms and personality.
7. Describe a store by its location and what it sells.
8. Describe a piece of jewelry by how it looks.
9. Describe a vegetable by some dishes in which this vegetable would be an ingredient.
10. Describe a city by the buildings and landmarks it has in it.
11. Describe a cartoon character by the characteristics and habits of the character.
12. Describe a song by its lyrics and tune.
13. Describe a person in history by why we remember the person.
14. Describe an individual sport (not team sport) by its rules.
15. Describe something you eat quite often.
16. Describe a magazine by the features it contains.
17. Describe a tool by how it looks.
18. Describe the outside of your home.
19. Describe someone you know by his or her personality.
20. Describe a theme park by its attractions.

Directions: Answer the question in detail.

1. Explain how to plant a small bush.
2. Explain how you play checkers.
3. Explain how to make a grilled cheese sandwich.
4. Explain how to get to the closest drugstore.
5. Explain how to check books out of the library.
6. Explain how to get money from an ATM machine.
7. Explain how to pay a bill by check.
8. Explain how to housebreak a puppy or train a kitten to a litter box.
9. Explain how to decide on whether to buy an insurance policy.
10. Explain how to decide when to discard items you no longer want.
11. Explain how to swim a certain stroke.
12. Explain how to make a bed.
13. Explain how to take care of a sprained ankle.
14. Explain how you pack a suitcase.
15. Explain what happened that caused you to be with me today.
16. Explain how you or someone in your family met his or her spouse.
17. Explain how to wash a load of laundry.
18. Explain how to take care of a cold.
19. Explain the importance of fiber in your diet.
20. Explain the meaning of life.

Directions: Talk about one of your favorite things and answer the question in detail.

1. Discuss a favorite movie. Include the stars, characters, a little bit about the story, and why you like it.
2. Discuss a favorite sport. Include how it became your favorite and how you play it.
3. Discuss a favorite food you make. Include the ingredients, how to prepare it, and how you came up with the recipe.
4. Discuss a favorite holiday. Include why you like it, what special things you do to celebrate, and any family traditions you have.
5. Discuss a very good friend. Include how and when you met the person and what makes this individual stand out from your other friends.
6. Discuss a favorite place to shop. Include its location, what you like about what it sells, and what you especially like to buy there and why.
7. Discuss a favorite male or female actor. Include a bit about the actor's different roles and rise to fame as well as why you particularly like this actor.
8. Discuss a favorite home you have lived in. Include what it looks like inside and out, when you lived there and why you like it.
9. Discuss a favorite comedian. Include some of the comedian's past accomplishments as well as why you find this person particularly funny.
10. Discuss a favorite dessert. Include how you make it or where you get it and why you like it so much.
11. Discuss a favorite guilty pleasure. This could be any type of guilty pleasure. Include why you chose the one you did, why there is guilt involved, and why it makes you feel so good.
12. Discuss a favorite article of clothing or piece of jewelry. Include when and where you got it, when you wore it if you don't wear it now, and why it is so special.
13. Discuss a favorite piece of furniture in your home. Include why you chose this piece, why it is your favorite, and where it is located.
14. Discuss a favorite place to go with friends. Include where the place is, who you like to go with, and why this is such a good place.
15. Discuss a favorite carryout place. Include the type of place it is, what else it offers, and what you usually order.
16. Discuss a favorite time of your day. Include when it is, why this time is so special, and what you usually do during the time.

17. Discuss a favorite car you have had or would like to have. Include when you had it, details about the car, and why you chose that car.

18. Discuss a favorite comfort food. Include details about the food, how you make it or where you get it, and what comfort it gives you.

19. Discuss a favorite outside activity. Include details about how and when to do the activity and any equipment that is needed for it.

20. Discuss a favorite type of reading material. Include why you like that type of material and give some examples of it.

Personal Topics

Directions: Answer the question in detail.

1. Who is the most unique person in your family and why?
2. If it applies, talk about the experience of the birth of your child or an animal.
3. Talk about a happy childhood memory.
4. What table manners were your parents strict about?
5. You have won $1,500,000 after taxes in the lottery. What would you do with the money?
6. What could you teach others that you have learned from your experiences?
7. Talk about a holiday tradition your family has.
8. When was the happiest time during your life and why?
9. What are or were your grandparents like?
10. What would you like to do but can't and never could.
11. Talk about traveling overseas. If you haven't, where would you like to go and why?
12. What are some of the best gifts you have received and why?
13. What do you remember about your year in first grade?
14. If you could, what would you write a book about and why? What type of book would it be?
15. Talk about a family gathering where everything seemed to go wrong.
16. What is the worst thing you ever got in trouble for?
17. Talk about someone you had to spend time with as a child but tried not to.
18. Talk about a good car trip and a bad car trip you had as a family.
19. When you were a child, what did you want to be when you grew up and why?
20. What were you afraid of as a child? Why, and has that changed?

Directions: Pretend you are in the situation that is given. Talk about how you would handle the situation and any questions you would ask or points you would make. Make up any details you need to make the situation more realistic.

1. How would you comfort a close friend whose engagement was just ended by the other person?
2. How would you decide what treatment to have if you were diagnosed with cancer?
3. How would you tell your boss you think some of his or her comments are offensive and that some of the things you are asked to do are inappropriate for the job?
4. How would you, as a physician, explain to a family that their loved one is dying?
5. How would you explain to a dedicated and hard-working player that he is cut from a team?
6. As a police officer, how would you confront parents who are having a party where underage drinking is occurring?
7. How would you explain to a client why his or her ideas for an ad campaign are terrible?
8. How would you explain to a valued employee that his or her job is being eliminated?
9. How would you handle the situation with a friend who is depressed and has hinted to you that life isn't worth it?
10. As a supervisor, how would you talk to a server about complaints from customers?
11. How would you convince a stubborn relative who has been drinking not to drive?
12. How would you defend a number of deductions you have taken on your tax returns?
13. As a boyfriend, how would you break up with a girl you have dated for two years?
14. As a teenager, how would you handle pressure to smoke?
15. How would you respond to people who are trying to convert you to their religious views?
16. How would you convince your spouse to give up smoking?
17. How would you handle your parent who is spoiling your child?
18. How would you convince an interviewer you are qualified for a job?
19. How would you confront a friend who you know is having an affair?
20. How would you react upon learning your antique is worth $90,000?

Directions: Take the role of the first person and explain how you would handle the situation.

1. a parent explaining the tooth fairy to a young child
2. a teenager convincing a father the new driver needs a car
3. a wife convincing a husband with high blood pressure to lose weight
4. a candidate for senator talking about local issues and asking for your vote
5. a young woman explaining to her boyfriend why she is saving herself for marriage
6. a cousin asking you to exaggerate his experience to help him get a job
7. a policeman informing a man that his wife is in the hospital following a serious accident
8. an adult child talking to a parent about why the parent needs to move into an assisted-care facility
9. a mother explaining to her four-year-old son he is going to have a baby sister or brother
10. a father trying to talk his daughter and her finacé into eloping in exchange for money
11. someone explaining what having a stroke / other medical problem is like
12. a husband telling his family that he has been laid off
13. parents discouraging a son from marrying someone they think is a loser
14. one spouse confronting the other about having an affair
15. a father convincing his 17-year-old who wants to drop out of high school the importance of a diploma
16. renters complaining to a landlord about the condition of their apartment building
17. a boss meeting with an employee about errors that have occurred in messages and bookkeeping
18. a married son explaining to his mother that he has made reservations for her to stay in a motel when she visits for a week
19. a teenager resisting peer pressure from friends to try drugs
20. an adult in his twenties telling his parents he is gay

Directions: Role-play the task as if you were in the situation. Tell about the planning, what you would do and details of the process. If appropriate, play the other person's role. Include at least three details or bits of information that can be answered with who, what, when, where, how, and why.

1. Make a doctor's appointment with a specialist you have never seen.
2. Order a full catered or carryout meal for six people.
3. Complain about your taxes at a local tax assessment meeting.
4. Have a conversation with someone who lives at least an hour away who you haven't seen in a long time.
5. Talk with a salesman about buying a used car and your options.
6. Strike up a conversation with a neighbor you don't talk to very much.
7. Plan a surprise party for someone you know.
8. Contact the police about some strange activities that you feel are happening.
9. Sell your car. Write an ad and give information to a caller about what a great deal it is.
10. Ask for a job change with reasons and ideas of what you would like to do. If you are not employed, discuss with your imaginary genie what you would like to do and how you would like to be paid.
11. Discuss things you would like to know about the life of a female relative who passed on before you got to know her.
12. You are receiving an award. Give your own introduction to the audience and talk about what the award is for and why you deserve it.
13. Choose one of your favorite stores. You are the customer consultant. Discuss changes that should be made to satisfy you. Include things such as inventory, business methods, redecorating, pricing, clerks. It is not your job to worry about the cost of your ideas.
14. Review a movie that you saw recently for a cable TV show.
15. You have one hour to address the U.S. Congress on domestic problems and on what issues you think their efforts and money should focus. Include one issue important in your state.
16. Discuss an idea you have for a movie. Tell about the story, how you came up with the idea and who you would want for the lead parts.
17. Make a three-minute dating video about yourself for a new dating service TV show.

18. Someone you admire very much is receiving an award. You have been asked to give a short speech about why you admire this person and how he or she has affected your life.

19. You are going to teach a community education class. Discuss the content and goals.

20. Your high school has asked you to be their next graduation speaker. Discuss what you will say including what thoughts you have looking back on your high school days.

Directions: Answer the question with yes or no and add at least two points that support your view.

1. Should smoking be banned from all public buildings?
2. Should there be caps on the salaries of professional athletes?
3. Should larger companies have stricter accounting practices?
4. Should those who drive without a license face stricter consequences?
5. Should senior citizens be given larger tax breaks?
6. Should expectant parents be required to take a parenting course?
7. Should America routinely send billions overseas to the governments of Third World countries?
8. Should taxes be raised on liquor and cigarettes?
9. Should adopted children be able to find out who their biological parents are?
10. Should convicted sex offenders be allowed to keep their past private?
11. Should people be allowed to protect their families or homes from harm using any means?
12. Should unions be mandatory at every larger worksite?
13. Should a high school diploma or its equivalent be the minimum job requirement for a job for anyone over the age of 19?
14. Should the government provide more help than it presently does to places ravaged by disasters?
15. Should there be stronger and more anti-pollution laws for companies?
16. Should people be allowed to purchase and take promising drugs before they are FDA-approved?
17. Should there be term limits on elected officials?
18. Should food product labels be more strictly coded?
19. Should it be made easier for victims of identity theft to clear their records?
20. Should correspondence on the Internet be more closely monitored—especially for children?

Directions: Explain whether you agree with the statement or not. Explain why you believe as you do and give examples.

1. Celebrities lose their privacy when they become famous.
2. Children who are spanked mind better than those who are not spanked.
3. Elected officials represent the views of the voters who elected them.
4. Cancer patients should not be told an estimated survival time.
5. Walking is the best exercise.
6. The millionaires of today grew up in wealthy families.
7. You are born with artistic ability; it cannot be learned.
8. Divorced people have better marriages the second time around.
9. There should be a national flat tax with no exceptions.
10. Bad news stories get more coverage than good news stories.
11. It is easy to change addictive behavior.
12. Just because a company goes bankrupt does not mean it had a bad product or service.
13. The winners of the medals are determined before the Olympic Games start.
14. The best vacations cost the least.
15. Everyone over the age of 21 should have a will.
16. Men are from Mars, women are from Venus.
17. A sense of humor will get you through tough times.
18. How you look on the outside is more important than who you are on the inside.
19. Fast food is not healthy food.
20. Unions are outdated and need to be eliminated or changed.

Directions: *Explain the controversy surrounding the issue. Give at least two statements supporting each side of the issue.*

1. capital punishment
2. marijuana for medicinal purposes
3. same-sex marriage
4. affirmative action
5. gun control
6. illegal immigrants
7. stock market
8. uniforms in public schools
9. laser eye surgery
10. bigamy
11. abortion
12. mandatory helmet and seat belt laws
13. wire-tapping
14. euthanasia
15. cosmetic surgery
16. official national language
17. space exploration program
18. child molesters
19. prenuptial agreement
20. genetic engineering (cloning)